Textbook for
CT-SCAN TECHNICIANS

*"Radiography is
where a picture is worth a thousand words
where capturing moments that change lives
where the image tells the story of health, hope, and healing."*
— ***Hariqbal Singh***

Textbook for
CT-SCAN TECHNICIANS

As per the Diploma and Certificate Courses on Radiography and CT-scan

Editor

Hariqbal Singh MD DMRD
Professor and Additional Director
Shrimati Kashibai Navale Medical College
Pune, Maharashtra, India

Foreword
ANV Prasad

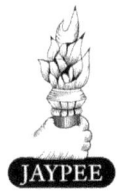

JAYPEE BROTHERS MEDICAL PUBLISHERS
The Health Sciences Publisher
New Delhi | London

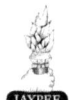 **Jaypee Brothers Medical Publishers (P) Ltd**

Headquarters
Jaypee Brothers Medical Publishers (P) Ltd
EMCA House, 23/23-B
Ansari Road, Daryaganj
New Delhi 110 002, India
Landline: +91-11-23272143, +91-11-23272703
+91-11-23282021, +91-11-23245672
Email: jaypee@jaypeebrothers.com

Corporate Office
Jaypee Brothers Medical Publishers (P) Ltd
4838/24, Ansari Road, Daryaganj
New Delhi 110 002, India
Phone: +91-11-43574357
Fax: +91-11-43574314
Email: jaypee@jaypeebrothers.com

Overseas Office
J.P. Medical Ltd
83 Victoria Street, London
SW1H 0HW (UK)
Phone: +44 20 3170 8910
Fax: +44 (0)20 3008 6180
Email: info@jpmedpub.com

Website: www.jaypeebrothers.com
Website: www.jaypeedigital.com

© 2024, Jaypee Brothers Medical Publishers

The views and opinions expressed in this book are solely those of the original contributor(s)/author(s) and do not necessarily represent those of editor(s) and publisher of the book.

All rights reserved. No part of this publication may be reproduced, stored or transmitted in any form or by any means, electronic, mechanical, photocopying, recording or otherwise, without the prior permission in writing of the publishers.

All brand names and product names used in this book are trade names, service marks, trademarks or registered trademarks of their respective owners. The publisher is not associated with any product or vendor mentioned in this book.

Medical knowledge and practice change constantly. This book is designed to provide accurate, authoritative information about the subject matter in question. However, readers are advised to check the most current information available on procedures included and check information from the manufacturer of each product to be administered, to verify the recommended dose, formula, method and duration of administration, adverse effects and contraindications. It is the responsibility of the practitioner to take all appropriate safety precautions. Neither the publisher nor the author(s)/editor(s) assume any liability for any injury and/or damage to persons or property arising from or related to use of material in this book.

This book is sold on the understanding that the publisher is not engaged in providing professional medical services. If such advice or services are required, the services of a competent medical professional should be sought.

Every effort has been made where necessary to contact holders of copyright to obtain permission to reproduce copyright material. If any have been inadvertently overlooked, the publisher will be pleased to make the necessary arrangements at the first opportunity.

Inquiries for bulk sales may be solicited at: jaypee@jaypeebrothers.com

Textbook for CT-Scan Technicians

First Edition: **2024**

ISBN: 978-93-5696-783-0

Dedicated to

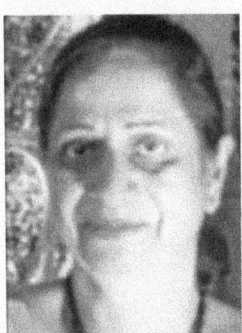

Arvind Hariqbal
My spouse, my confidante, muse, friend, and supporter,
who has been my profound inspiration.

Foreword

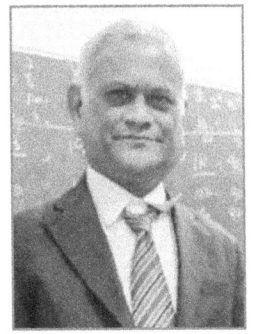

"Beauty is the reality that can be seen through the eyes of love." Brig Dr Hariqbal Singh is an exceptional teacher and inspiring guide to all. I greatly admire and adore him as the Veda Vyasa of Radiology for his expertise and masterful approach to simply presenting complex knowledge.

The present *Textbook for CT-Scan Technicians* is a wonderful contribution to the field of imaging technology. It covers from basic anatomy to technological advancements.

The book's lucid presentation and illustrations make it an excellent resource for students and teaching faculty of imaging technology. It is a must-have for every medical college library.

With the help of this marvelous book, students of all levels of medical imaging technology can excel in performance with confidence.

ANV Prasad
MD DMRD DIH DPPH MA PhD
Professor and Head of Radiology
Sri Madhusudan Sai Institute of Medical Sciences
Karnataka, India

Preface

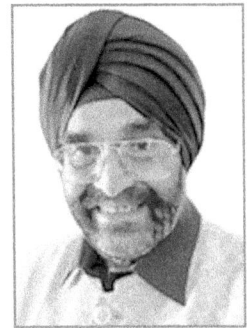

It was purely a contemplation of Shri Jitendar P Vij, Group Chairman, Jaypee Brothers Medical Publishers (P) Ltd., as the need of the hour and trust that led to development of this book.

Technician is a skilled person trained in operation of CT equipment, its technicalities, and safety compliance. This book is designed for the innovative and fresh CT technologist and the one already trained, and those interested in performing CT.

Since inception of CT in early 1970s, it has made an enormous impact in diagnostic imaging. Over the years, improvements in both CT hardware and software have resulted in advances in all its major features including image resolution and reconstruction speed. For this, well-qualified technicians are the requirement of the day.

Cross-sectional anatomy forms a very important part of training. Anatomy makes the technologist know as to what he is dealing with. Anatomy forms a strong base for CT technicians.

The complex physics component is presented in a simple understandable language. It covers all technical details pertaining to CT scan with illustrations.

This is an excellent book for students and teachers practicing the art and science of computed tomography.

Hariqbal Singh

Acknowledgments

I thank Dr Arvind V Bhore, Director, Shrimati Kashibai Navale Medical College, Pune, Maharashtra, India for his kind acquiescence in this endeavor.

My extraordinary thanks to Dr Prashant Naik and postgraduate trainees Dr Loobina Kodnani, Shreyash Bhoyar, Gayatri Chaphalkar and Ram Rathod for checking the manuscript.

My incredible thanks to the consultants Dr Santosh Konde, Sasane Amol, Pooja Shah, Yasmeen Khan, Vivek Choudhari, and Varsha Sonawane who have helped in congregation of required imagery.

Very special appreciation to the technicians Rahul More and Mritunjoy Srivastava for their untiring help in retrieving data.

My appreciation and gratitude to Snehal Bhairamadgikar and Shrikant Adat for their constant secretarial assistance.

I am also indebted to Shri Jitendar P Vij (Group Chairman), Mr Ankit Vij (Managing Director), Mr MS Mani (Group President), Dr Madhu Choudhary (Director—Educational Publishing), Ms Pooja Bhandari [Director-Production (Books and Journals)], Ms Sunita Katla (EA to Group Chairman and Publishing Manager), Ms Samina Khan (EA to Director—Educational Publishing), Dr Upma Tomar (Development Editor), Mr Ajay Kumar Sharma [DGM (Books and Journals)], Mr Rajesh Sharma (Production Coordinator), Ms Seema Dogra (Cover Visualizer), Ms Neha Verma (Graphic Designer), Ms Neelam Kakriya (Proofreader), Mr Kulwant Singh (Typesetter), and Mr Radhe Shyam (Graphic Designer) who involved in the production process.

Last but not least, I am grateful to God and mankind who have allowed me for this wonderful experience.

Contents

SECTION 1: CROSS-SECTIONAL ANATOMY ON CT SCAN

Chapter 1:	Anatomical Planes	3
Chapter 2:	Brain and Orbit	5
Chapter 3:	Temporal Bone	16
Chapter 4:	Paranasal Sinuses	19
Chapter 5:	Face and Neck	24
Chapter 6:	Vertebral Column	29
Chapter 7:	Chest and Mediastinum	37
Chapter 8:	Heart	46
Chapter 9:	Abdomen and Pelvis	50
Chapter 10:	Joints of Upper Extremity	64
Chapter 11:	Joints of Lower Extremity	76

SECTION 2: EQUIPMENT, PHYSICS AND PROCEDURES

Chapter 12:	Radiography and the Radiographer	87
Chapter 13:	The CT Technologist	88
Chapter 14:	Artificial Intelligence on CT Imaging	89
Chapter 15:	AERB Requirements for Installation of CT Scan	90
Chapter 16:	Production of X-rays	91
Chapter 17:	Generations of CT System	93
Chapter 18:	Collimators and Filtration	99
Chapter 19:	Components of CT Scanner	100
Chapter 20:	Hounsfield Scale	104
Chapter 21:	Image Reconstruction	106
Chapter 22:	Window Setting	107
Chapter 23:	Three-Dimensional Imaging	109
Chapter 24:	Volumetric Rendering Techniques	110
Chapter 25:	CT Fluoroscopy	113
Chapter 26:	CT Contrast	114
Chapter 27:	CT Myelography	120
Chapter 28:	CT Angiography	121

Chapter 29:	Artifacts	123
Chapter 30:	Thermoluminescent Dosimeter	126
Chapter 31:	Diagnosis on CT Images	128
Chapter 32:	Interventional Radiology	132
Chapter 33:	Tidbits on CT Scan	136
Chapter 34:	CT Scan versus MRI Scan	138
Chapter 35:	Medical Records	139
Chapter 36:	Radiation Units	140
Chapter 37:	Radiation Hazards	141
Chapter 38:	Radiation Protection	143
Chapter 39:	Picture Archiving and Communication System	147
Chapter 40:	Cloud Computing	153
Chapter 41:	Photon-Counting Detector CT	154
Chapter 42:	CT Technologist Questions/Answers	155

Index   *159*

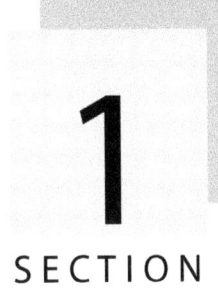

SECTION 1

CROSS-SECTIONAL ANATOMY ON CT SCAN

SECTION OUTLINE

- **Chapter 1:** Anatomical Planes
- **Chapter 2:** Brain and Orbit
- **Chapter 3:** Temporal Bone
- **Chapter 4:** Paranasal Sinuses
- **Chapter 5:** Face and Neck
- **Chapter 6:** Vertebral Column
- **Chapter 7:** Chest and Mediastinum
- **Chapter 8:** Heart
- **Chapter 9:** Abdomen and Pelvis
- **Chapter 10:** Joints of Upper Extremity
- **Chapter 11:** Joints of Lower Extremity

CHAPTER 1

Anatomical Planes

The anatomical planes are used to describe the location of structures in human anatomy. The planes used are—transverse or axial, sagittal and coronal (**Fig. 1**).

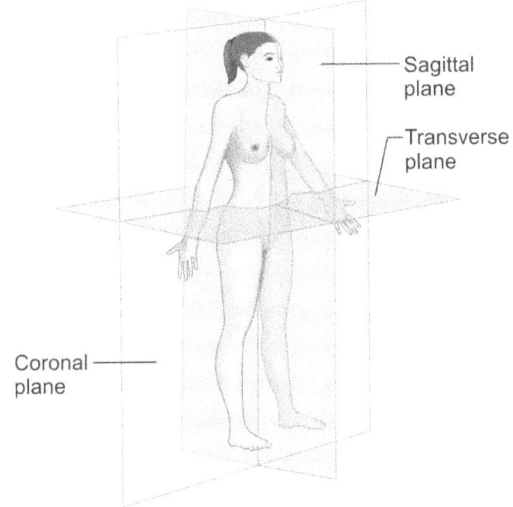

Fig. 1: Showing axial, sagittal and coronal planes.

TRANSVERSE OR AXIAL PLANE (FIG. 2A)

The axial plane is a horizontal plane. It is perpendicular to both the sagittal and coronal planes, and parallel to the ground. It divides the body into an upper (superior) section and a lower (inferior) section.

SAGITTAL PLANE (FIG. 2B)

The sagittal plane is a vertical plane which passes through the body longitudinally. It divides the body into left and right section, median sagittal plane passes down the midline of the body.

CORONAL PLANE (FIG. 2C)

The coronal plane is a vertical plane which passes through the body longitudinally—but perpendicular to the sagittal plane. It divides the body into a front (anterior) section and back (posterior) section.

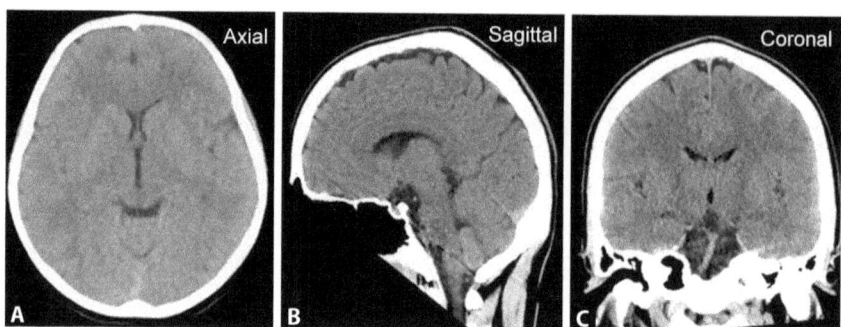

Figs. 2A to C: CT scan of brain, showing the three anatomical planes: Axial, Sagittal and Coronal.

CHAPTER 2

Brain and Orbit

Brain is enclosed in the cranium which includes all the bones that make the skeleton of head and are joined to each other with help of joints known as sutures. Inner part of skull base is divided into anterior, middle and posterior cranial fossae.

Skull base has multiple foramen through which various nerves and vessels pass.

Foramen rotundum is situated in greater wing of sphenoid, it connects middle cranial fossa and pterygopalatine fossa. Maxillary division of trigeminal nerve, artery of foramen rotundum and an emissary vein pass through it.

Foramen lacerum is located at lower aspect of medial pterygoid plate. Nerve to pterygoid canal and meningeal branch of ascending pharyngeal artery pass through it.

Foramen spinosum is situated in greater wing of sphenoid posterolateral to foramen ovale. Middle meningeal artery, vein and lesser superficial petrosal nerve and meningeal branch of mandibular nerve pass through it.

Foramen ovale connects infratemporal fossa and middle cranial fossa. Mandibular division of trigeminal nerve, lesser petrosal nerve, accessory meningeal artery and emissary vein pass through it.

Foramen magnum is located in the occipital bone. It contains medulla oblongata, spinal accessory nerve, vertebral artery and spinal arteries.

Jugular foramen is located at posterior end of petro-occipital suture. Inferior petrosal sinus, meningeal branches of pharyngeal artery and occipital artery pass through its anterior part. IXth, Xth and XIth cranial nerves pass through its intermediate part. Internal jugular vein is located in its posterior most part.

Orbitomeatal line is an imaginary line running from external auditory meatus to superior wall of orbit. Sections of CT scan of brain are taken parallel to this line.

Embryologically brain develops from neural plate which arises from the ectoderm on dorsal aspect of embryo at around 4-5 weeks of intrauterine life. Maximum growth occurs in the second trimester. Pattern of myelination extends caudocranially and posteroanteriorly.

Anatomically brain is divided into forebrain (prosencephalon), midbrain (mesencephalon) and hindbrain (rhombencephalon).

Forebrain (prosencephalon) consists of:
- Cerebrum (telencephalon) includes cerebral hemispheres, caudate nucleus and putamen.
- Diencephalon includes epithalamus (pineal gland), thalamus, hypothalamus and globus pallidus.

Midbrain (mesencephalon): It consist of corpora quadrigemina, tectum, cerebral peduncles and suprapontine portion.

Hindbrain (rhombencephalon) consists of:
- Metencephalon which includes cerebellar hemispheres and the vermis.
- Myelencephalon made of pons and medulla oblongata.

Brainstem is composed of mesencephalon and myelencephalon. Cranial nerve nuclei are located in the brainstem.

The cross-section of head shows **(Figs. 1 to 14):**

- ❖ Scalp has five layers from outside inwards: skin, subcutaneous fibro-adipose layer, galea aponeurotica, subgaleal areolar tissue layer and pericranium.
- ❖ Calvarium or skull table which includes inner and outer tables of bones. Outer table is made of strong compact bone. Inner table has thin brittle compact bone. Diplopic space between these two skull tables is made of trabecular bone and is filled by red marrow.
- ❖ Meninges of the brain include the outer pachymeninges (dura mater) and inner leptomeninges (arachnoid and pia mater).
- ❖ Subperiosteal space is between calvarium and periosteum of outer skull table. Bleeding here leads to cephalohematoma.
- ❖ Epidural or extradural space is between periosteum of inner skull table and calvarium.
- ❖ Subdural space is within inner layer of dura and arachnoid mater. Subarachnoid space exists between arachnoid and pia mater. Subpial space is the perivascular Virchow-Robin space that exists in brain.
- ❖ Cerebrospinal fluid fills the entire ventricular system, sulci and cisterns. There is 150 mL of total CSF in an adult. It is produced at the rate of 0.4 mL/min by choroid plexuses in the lateral ventricles. The flow is as follows:

  From lateral ventricles it enters the third ventricle via foramen of Monro. From third ventricle it goes through aqueduct of Sylvius and enters the fourth ventricle. Foramen of Luschka and foramen of Magendie are the outlets of CSF from fourth ventricle to various sulci and cisterns surrounding brain. From these sulci and cisterns CSF is absorbed in the venous system through arachnoid villae. Small amount also continues into the CSF filled spinal canal located at center of spinal cord.
- ❖ Each part of brain has an outer grey matter (collection of nerve cells) and an inner white matter (nerve fibers and tracts).
- ❖ Basal ganglia is a group of neurons lying deep within the cortex. Basal ganglia consists of claustrum, corpus striatum [caudate + lentiform nucleus (putamen and globus pallidus)] and amygdaloid body.
- ❖ Pituitary gland is located in the pituitary fossa of sphenoid bone, the roof of which is formed by diaphragma sellae. Pituitary gland has an anterior lobe, pars intermedia and a posterior lobe.
- ❖ Brain is supplied by carotid and vertebral arteries. Common carotid artery divides into the internal carotid artery and external carotid artery. Internal carotid artery supplies the brain. It has cervical, petrous, cavernous and supraclinoid segments. Supraclinoid segment gives rise to anterior and middle cerebral arteries. Posterior cerebral artery arises from basilar artery which is formed after fusion of vertebral arteries.

  The arterial anastomoses of the brain is called circle of Willis which is contributed by the anterior, middle and posterior cerebral arteries to supply blood to entire brain.

  Cerebellum is supplied by anterior and posterior inferior cerebellar arteries and superior cerebellar arteries which arise from vertebrobasilar arteries which originates from subclavian artery or directly from aorta.

  Various veins collect the blood from brain and drain into venous sinuses which drain into the internal jugular vein.

Note: *With each image the topogram shows the level of the section which enhances the understanding of anatomy. Recon is reconstruction.*

Chapter 2: Brain and Orbit

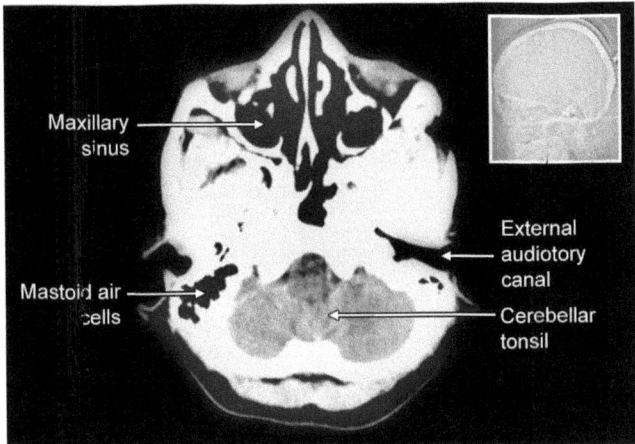

Fig. 1: Axial CT section of brain at the level of cerebellum.

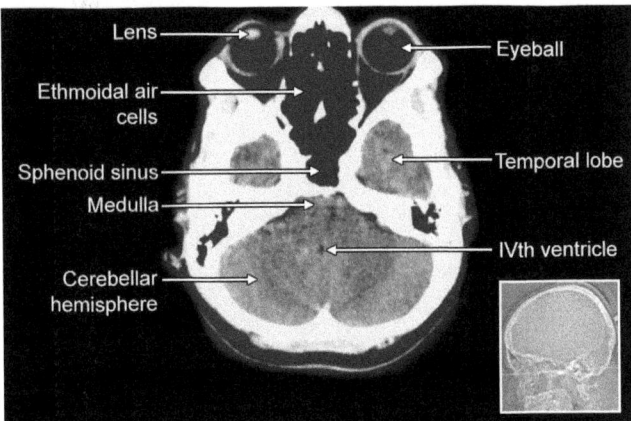

Fig. 2: Axial CT section of brain at the level of IVth ventricle.

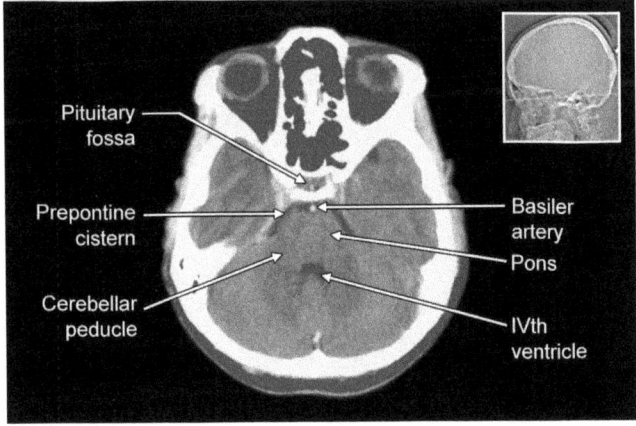

Fig. 3: Axial CT section of brain at the level of pituitary gland.

Section 1: Cross-Sectional Anatomy on CT Scan

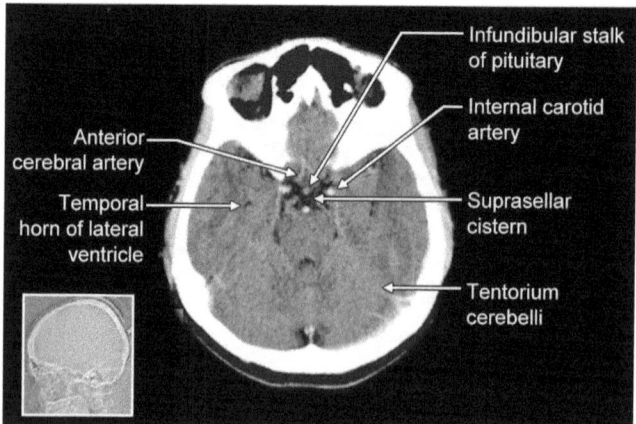

Fig. 4: Axial CT section of brain at the level of temporal lobes.

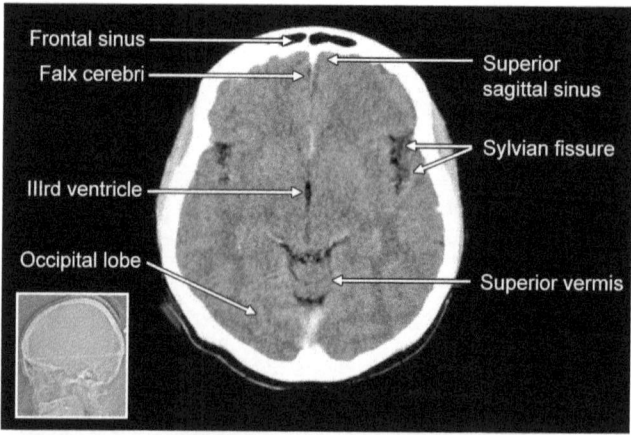

Fig. 5: Axial CT section of brain at the level of IIIrd ventricle.

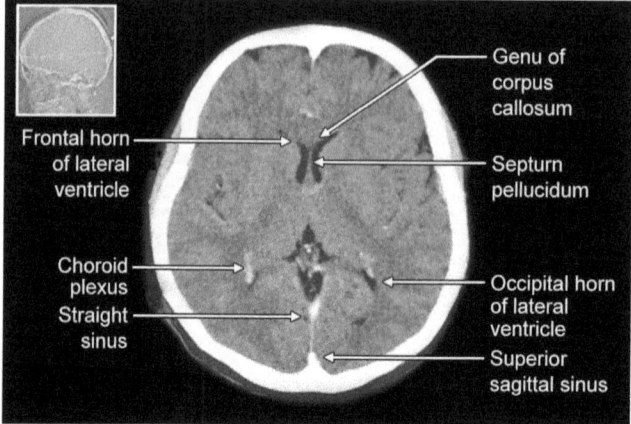

Fig. 6: Axial CT section of brain at the level of lateral ventricles.

Chapter 2: Brain and Orbit

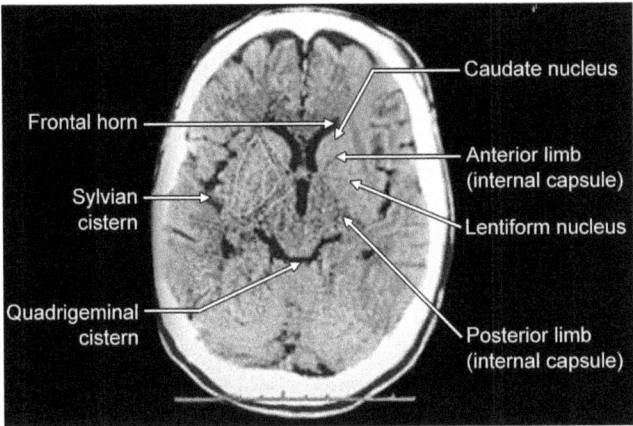

Fig. 7: Axial CT section of brain at the level of basal ganglion.

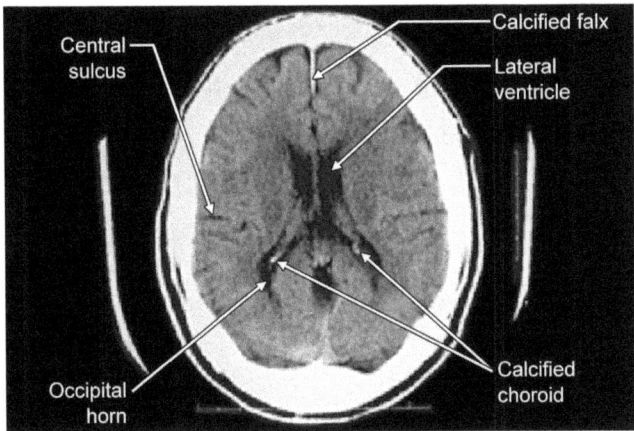

Fig. 8: Axial CT section of brain at the level of entire cerebral hemisphere.

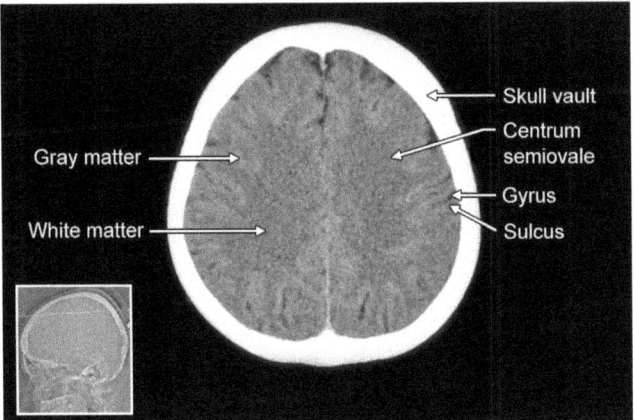

Fig. 9: Axial CT section of brain at the level of centrum semiovale.

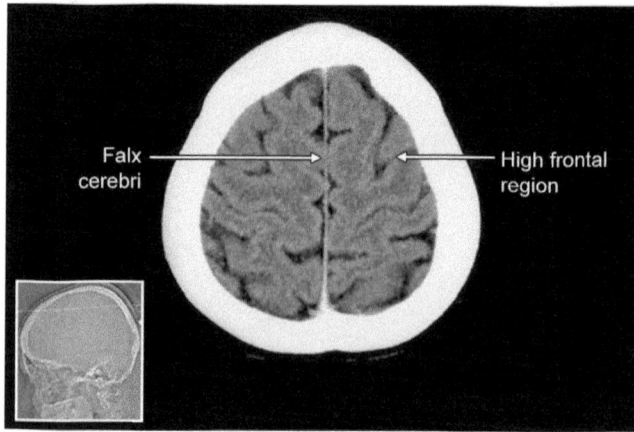

Fig. 10: Axial CT section of brain showing high frontal lobe.

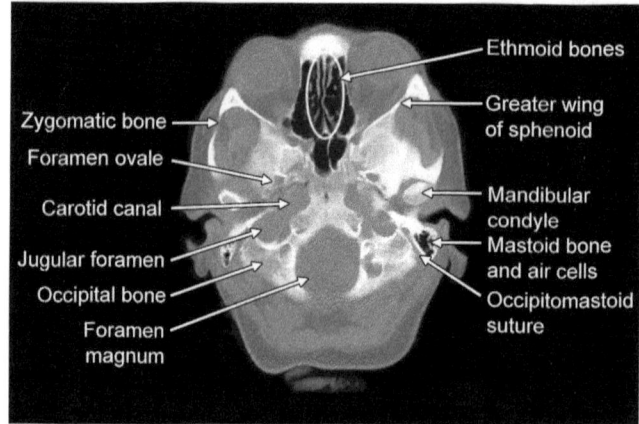

Fig. 11: Axial CT section of brain at the level of bas of skull.

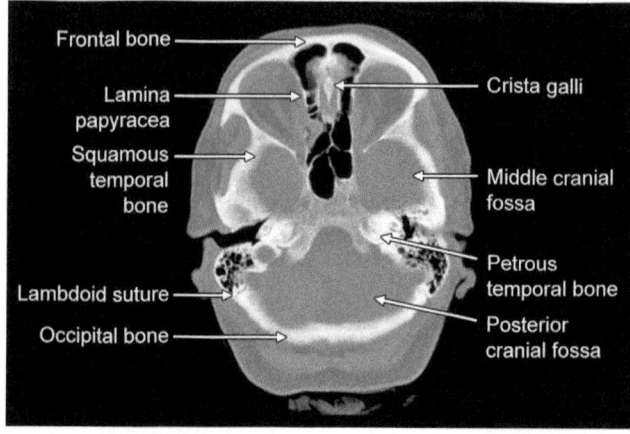

Fig. 12: Axial CT section of head in bone window.

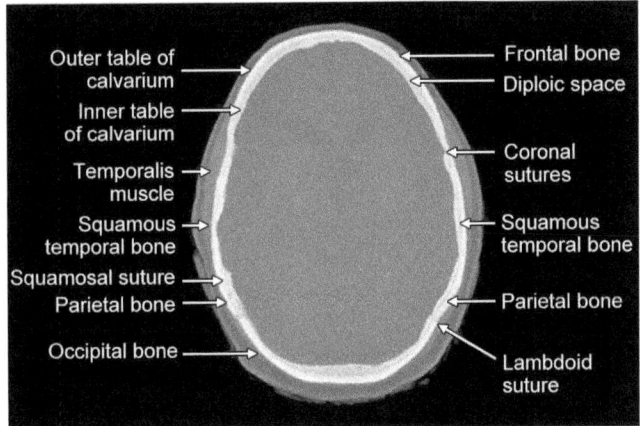

Fig. 13: Axial CT section of head in bone window showing all bones of vault of skull.

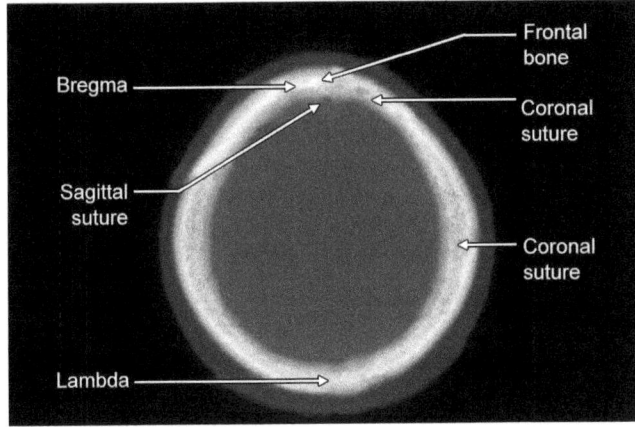

Fig. 14: Axial CT section of head in bone window showing high frontal bone.

CIRCLE OF WILLIS

The circle of Willis is a ring of vessels connecting the anterior and posterior circulations of the brain **(Fig. 15)**. The ring is bounded anteriorly by a single anterior communicating artery (ACom), which connects the bilateral anterior cerebral arteries (ACA).

Arteries forming circle of Willis are:
- Anterior cerebral artery (left and right) at their A1 segments.
- Anterior communicating artery.
- Internal carotid artery (left and right) at its distal tip (carotid terminus).
- Posterior cerebral artery (left and right) at their P1 segments.
- Posterior communicating artery (left and right).

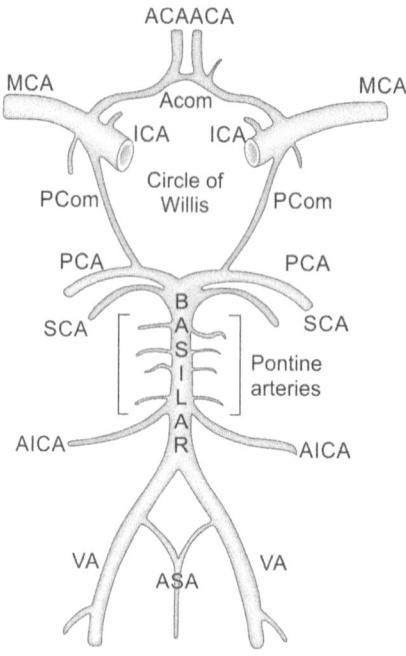

Fig. 15: Circle of Willis.
(ACA: Anterior cerebral artery; A Com: Anterior communicating artery; MCA: Middle cerebral artery; ICA–Internal carotid artery; PCom: Posterior communicating artery; PCA: Posterior cerebral artery; SCA: Superior cerebellar artery; BASILAR: Basilar artery; AICA: Anterior inferior cerebellar artery; VA: Vertebral artery; ASA: Anterior spinal artery)

ORBIT

Orbit is a pyramid-shaped cavity. Roof of orbit is formed by orbital plate of the frontal bone. Medial wall is the thinnest and is formed by a small portion of the frontal process of maxilla, lacrimal bone, ethmoid bone and body of sphenoid. Floor is made by the orbital part of maxillary bone. Lateral orbital wall is the thickest and is formed by orbital surface of the greater wing of sphenoid **(Figs. 16 to 23)**. Eyeball is the main structure of the anterior orbit; it is divided into small anterior chamber and larger posterior chamber (vitreous), by the lens.

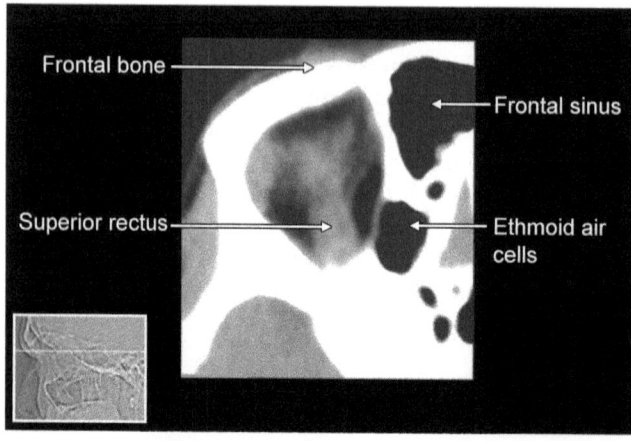

Fig. 16: Axial CT section of right orbit.

Chapter 2: Brain and Orbit

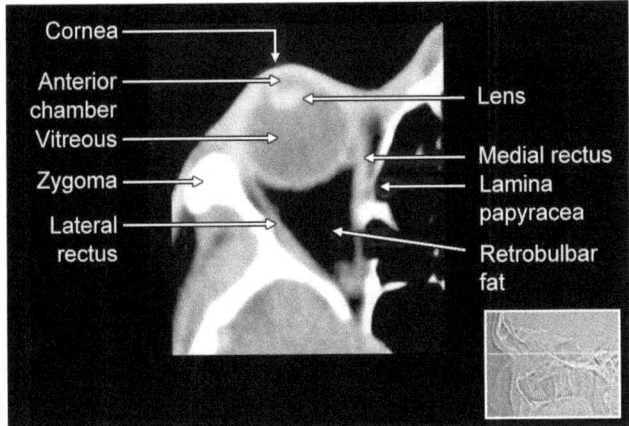

Fig. 17: Axial CT section of right orbit.

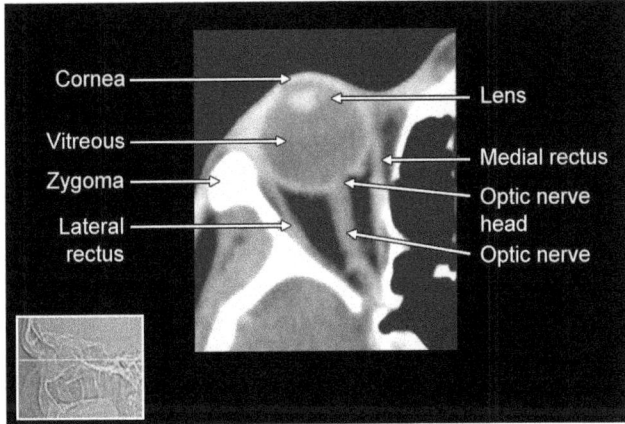

Fig. 18: Axial CT section of right orbit.

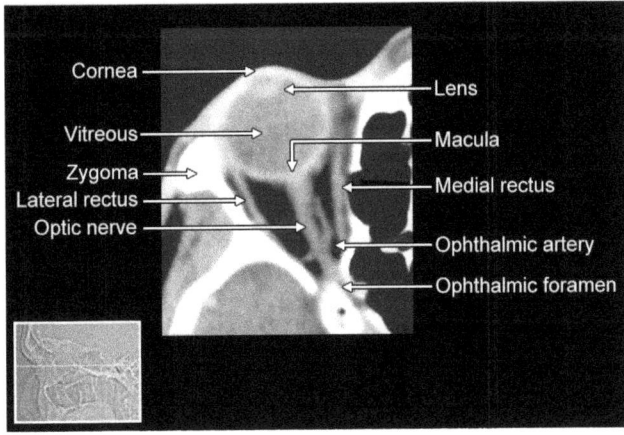

Fig. 19: Axial CT section of right orbit.

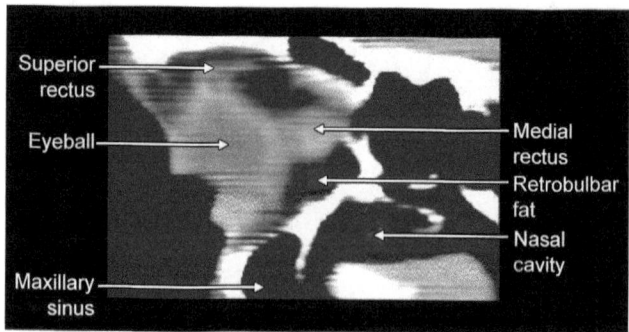

Fig. 20: Sagittal CT recon of right orbit.

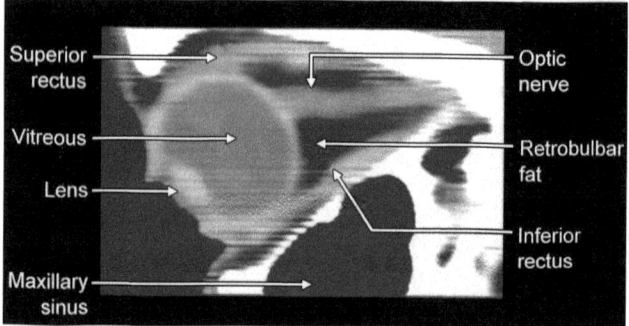

Fig. 21: Sagittal CT recon of right orbit.

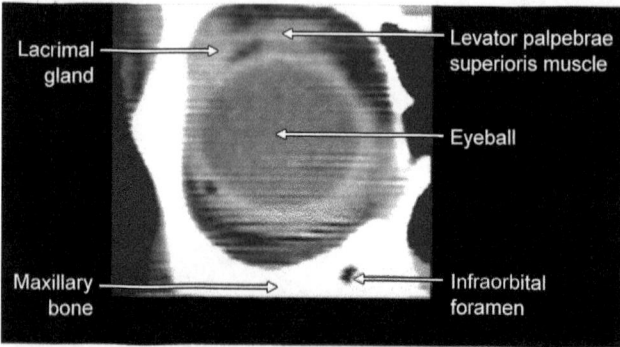

Fig. 22: Coronal CT recon of right orbit.

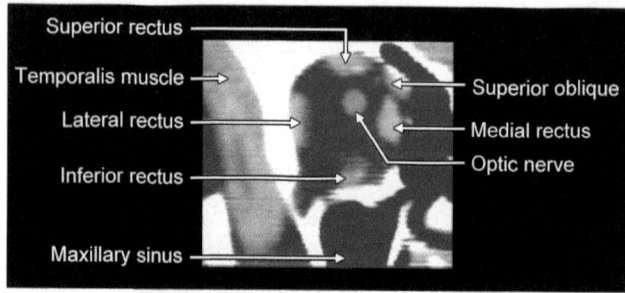

Fig. 23: Coronal CT recon of right orbit.

Optic nerve along with ophthalmic artery passes posteriorly into the middle cranial fossa through the optic canal. Superior orbital fissure is present between the greater and lesser wings of sphenoid. Oculomotor, trochlear and abducent nerves (III, IV and VI cranial nerves), lacrimal, frontal and nasal branches of the trigeminal nerve, ophthalmic veins and anterior connections between the middle meningeal and ophthlamic artery passes through the superior orbital fissure. Inferior orbital fissure lies between the lateral and inferior orbital walls and emissary veins pass through it.

CHAPTER 3

Temporal Bone

Temporal bone (Figs. 1 to 8) has following parts:
1. Squamous
2. Mastoid
3. Petrous
4. Tympanic
5. Styloid

Ear is divided into external ear, middle ear and inner ear.

External ear has a bony and a cartilaginous external auditory canal and extends medially upto tympanic membrane **(Fig. 1)**.

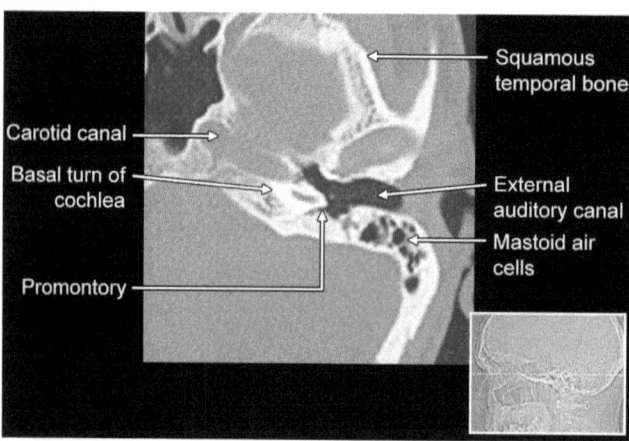

Fig. 1: Axial CT section of left temporal bone.

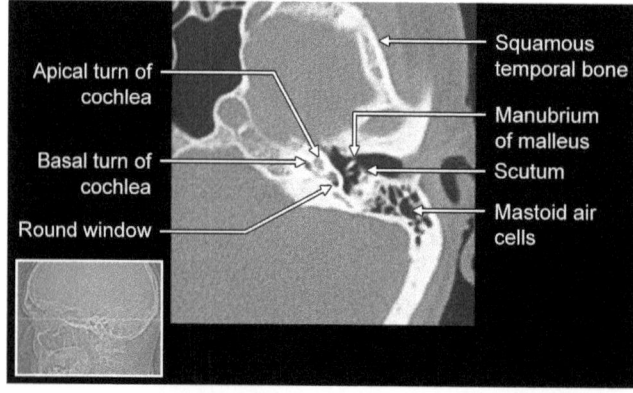

Fig. 2: Axial CT section of left temporal bone.

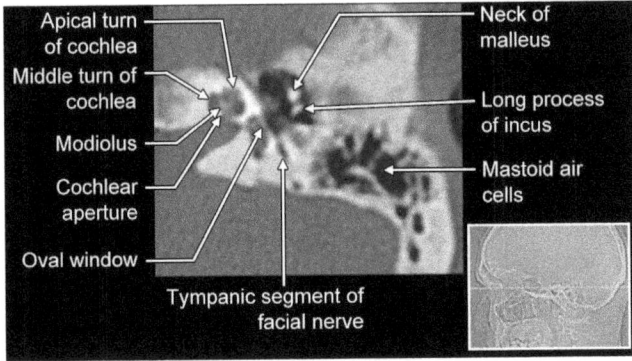

Fig. 3: Axial CT section of left temporal bone.

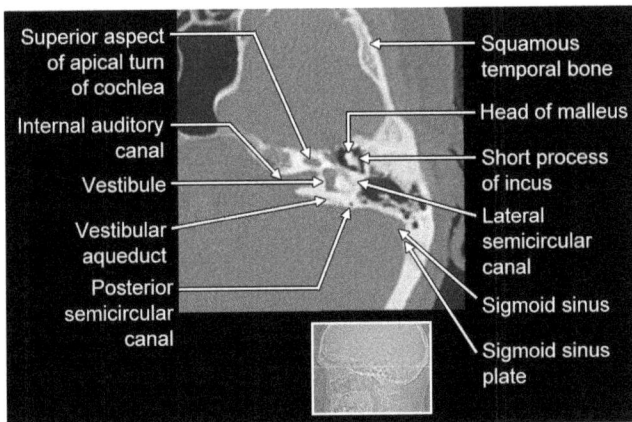

Fig. 4: Axial CT section of left temporal bone.

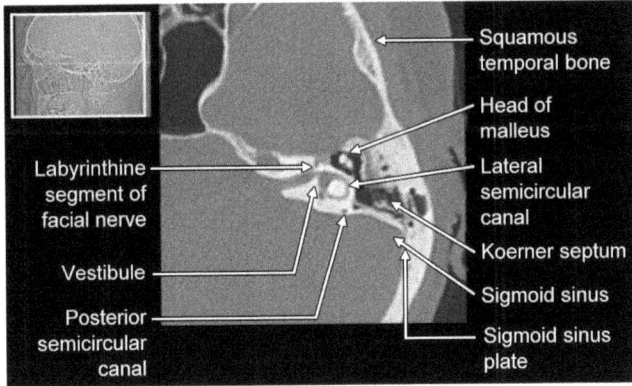

Fig. 5: Axial CT section of left temporal bone.

Middle ear extends from tympanic membrane to the wall of bony labyrinth. It is divided into epitympanum, mesotympanum and hypotympanum by an upper line passing through inferior tip of scutum and a lower line drawn parallel to inferior aspect of bony external auditory canal. The auditory ossicles are—malleus, incus and stapes.

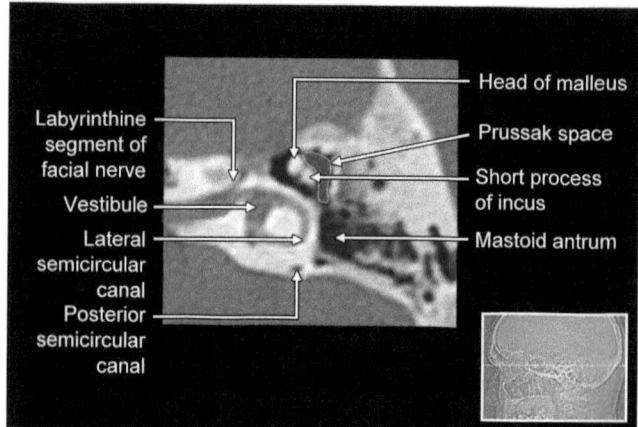

Fig. 6: Axial CT section of left temporal bone magnified view.

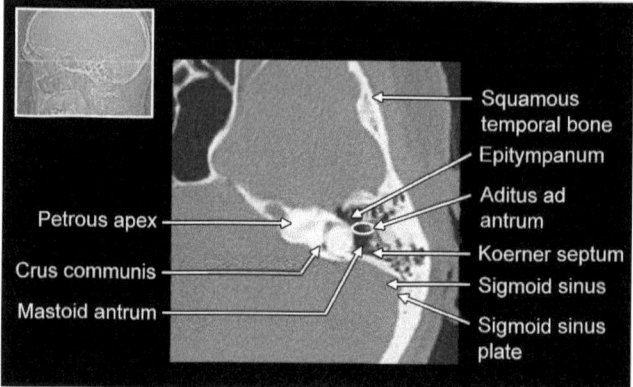

Fig. 7: Axial CT section of left temporal bone.

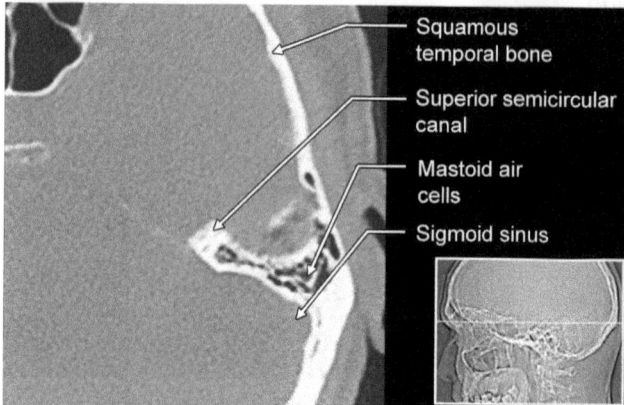

Fig. 8: Axial CT section of left temporal bone.

Inner ear includes the two and half turns of cochlea, vestibule, semicircular canals, cochlear aqueduct and vestibular aqueduct.

CHAPTER 4

Paranasal Sinuses

Paranasal sinuses include maxillary sinuses, frontal sinus, anterior and posterior ethmoid sinuses and sphenoid sinus **(Figs. 1 to 13)**. They are lined with mucous membrane and communicate with nasal cavity.

Ostiomeatal unit (OMU) is the common drainage for frontal, maxillary and anterior and middle ethmoid air cells into the nose. It produces two liters of mucus per day which travels towards nasopharynx at the rate of 1 cm/minute.

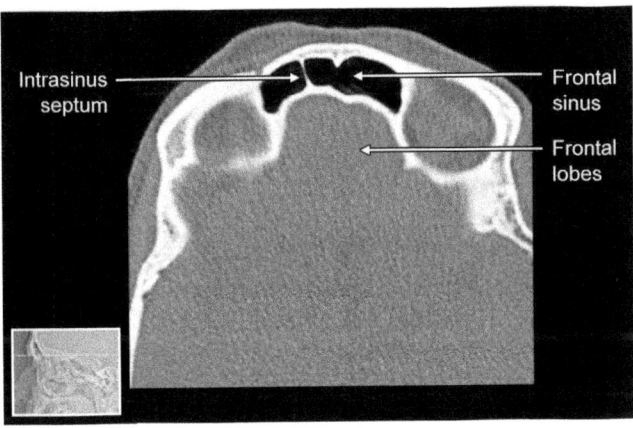

Fig. 1: Axial CT section of PNS.

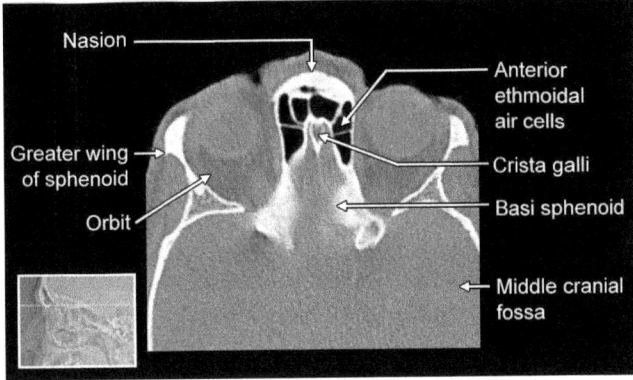

Fig. 2: Axial CT section of PNS.

Section 1: Cross-Sectional Anatomy on CT Scan

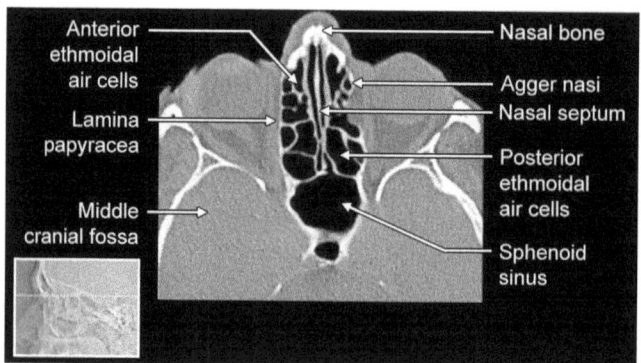

Fig. 3: Axial CT section of PNS.

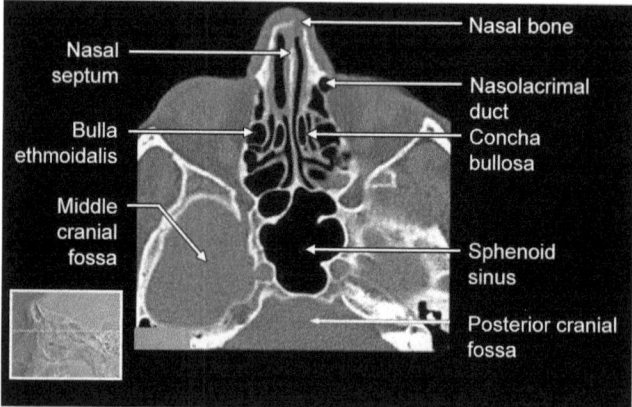

Fig. 4: Axial CT section of PNS.

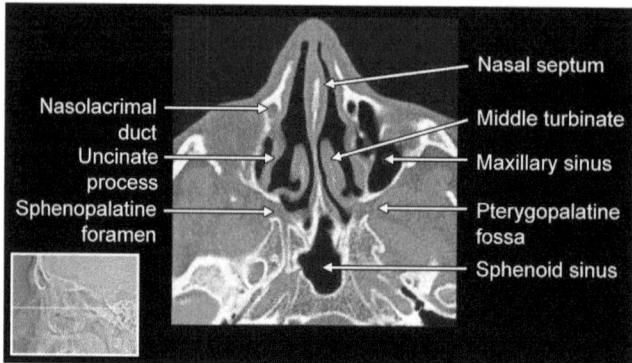

Fig. 5: Axial CT section of PNS.

Chapter 4: Paranasal Sinuses

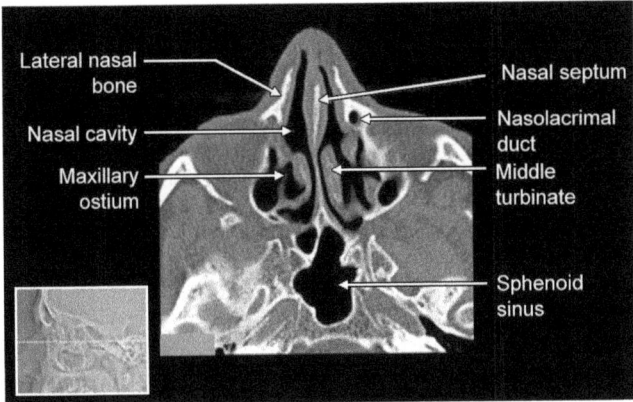

Fig. 6: Axial CT section of PNS.

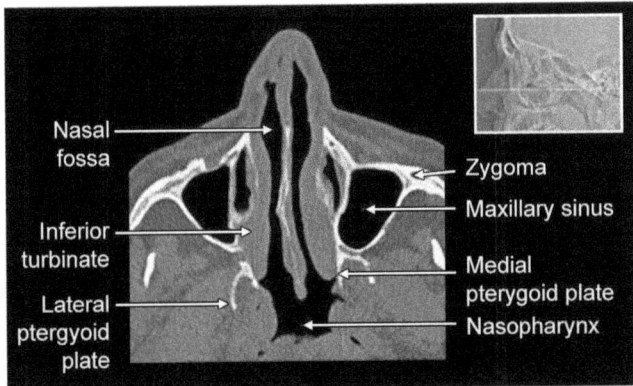

Fig. 7: Axial CT section of PNS.

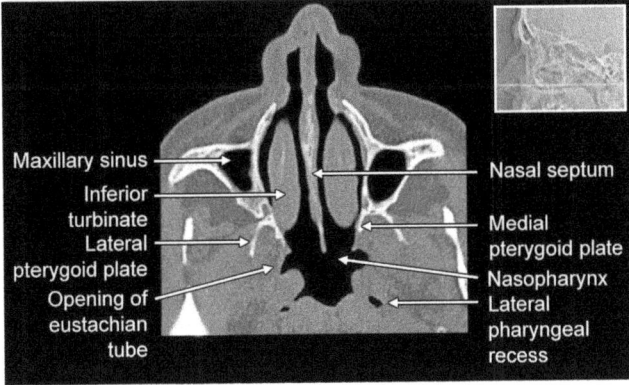

Fig. 8: Axial CT section of PNS.

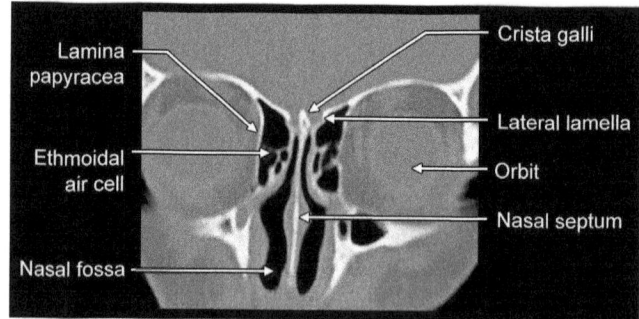

Fig. 9: Coronal CT recon of PNS.

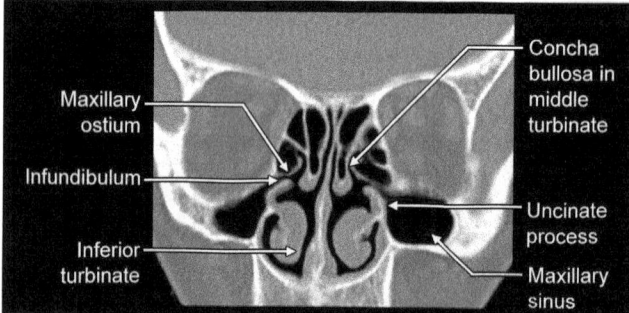

Fig. 10: Coronal CT recon of PNS.

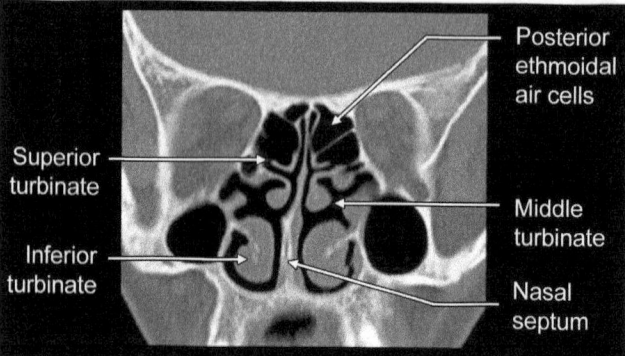

Fig. 11: Coronal CT recon of PNS.

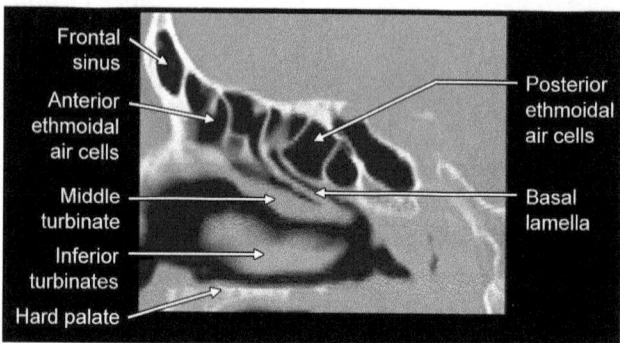

Fig. 12: Sagittal CT recon of PNS.

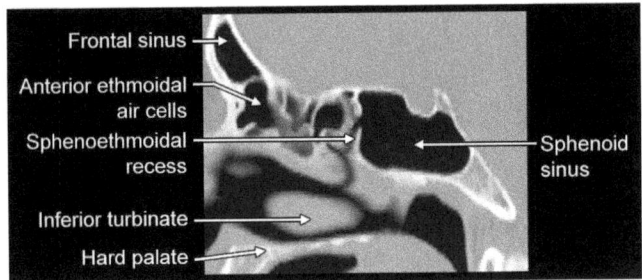

Fig. 13: Sagittal CT reconstruction of PNS.

Certain variants of ethmoidal air cells are:
- **Onodi cells:** Pneumatized posterior most ethmoid air cells extending into sphenoid bone and optic canal.
- **Ethmoid bulla:** Air cell posterosuperior to infundibulum and lateral to lamina papyracea.
- **Haller cell** is inferolateral to ethmoid bulla and protrudes into maxillary sinus.
- **Agger nasi** is the anterior most air cell in front of attachment of middle turbinate to cribriform plate.

Face and Neck

CHAPTER 5

Oral cavity includes lip, gingiva, buccal mucosa, hard palate, floor of mouth and anterior two-thirds of tongue (**Figs. 1 to 5**). Oropharynx includes pharyngeal wall between nasopharynx and pharyngoepiglottic fold, soft palate, tonsillar region and the base of tongue.

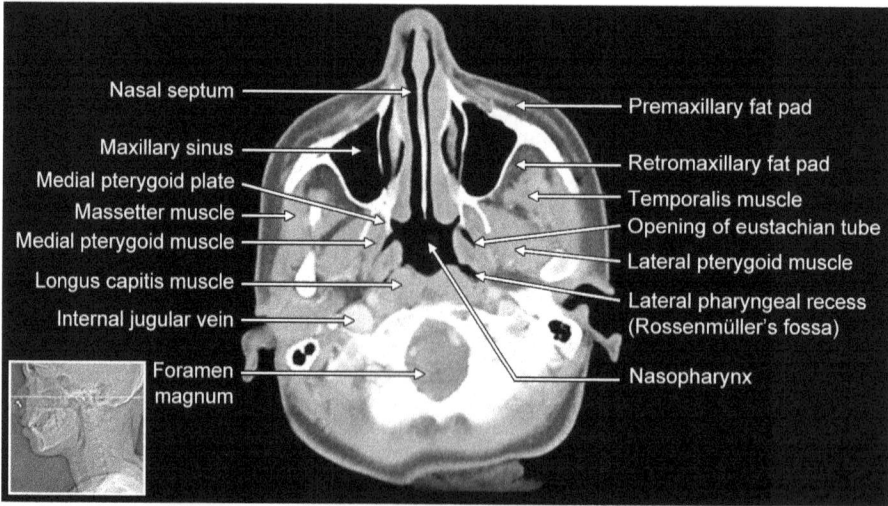

Fig. 1: Axial CT section of neck—level maxillary sinuses.

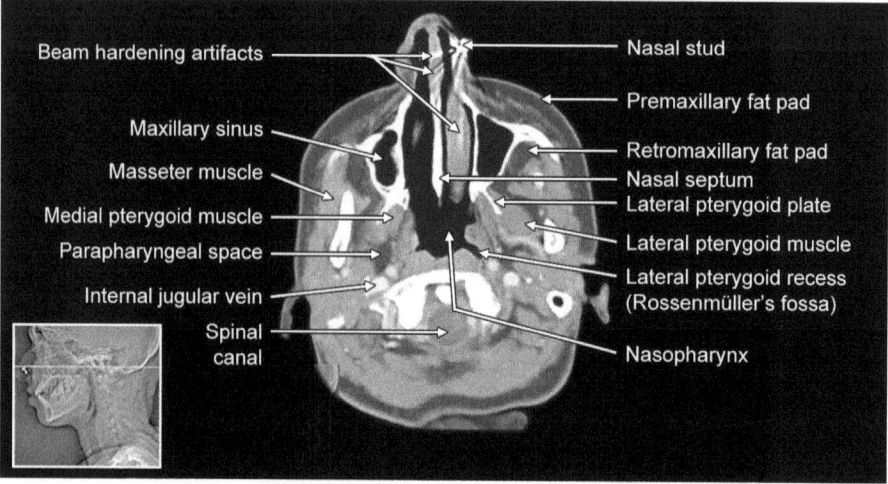

Fig. 2: Axial CT section of neck—level superior part of maxillary sinuses.

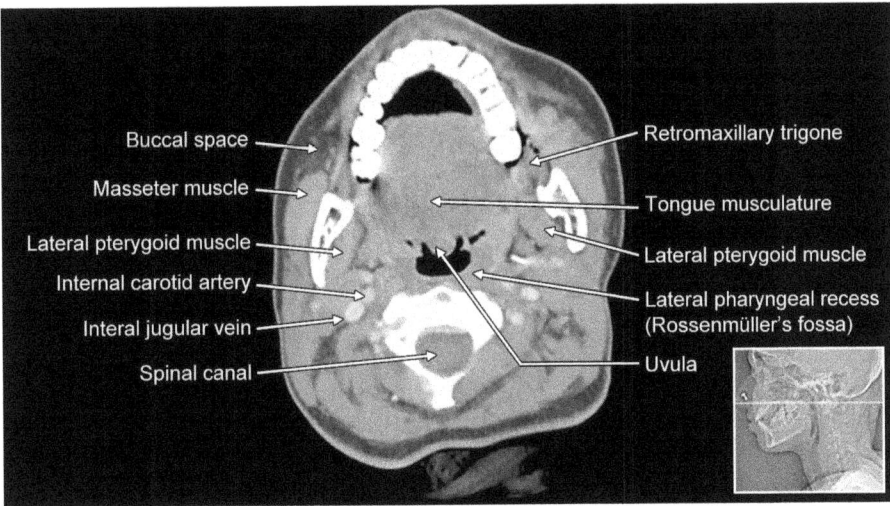

Fig. 3: Axial CT section of neck—level uvula.

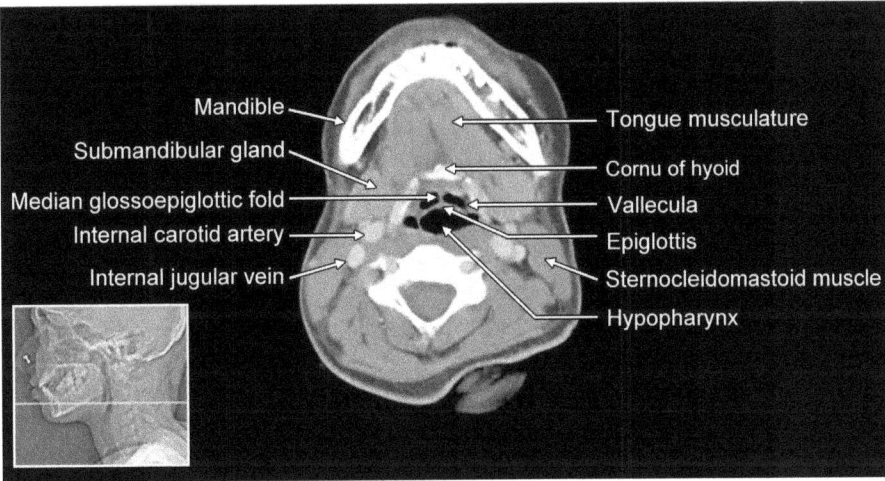

Fig. 4: Axial CT section of neck—level epiglottis.

Hypopharynx is the aerodigestive tract between hyoid bone and inferior aspect of the cricoid cartilage **(Figs. 5 and 6)**. It includes pyriform sinuses, pharyngoesophageal junction and posterior hypopharyngeal wall from valleculae to cricoarytenoid joints.

Larynx includes supraglottic, glottic and subglottic compartments **(Figs. 7 to 10)**. Supraglottic compartment is from tongue base and valleculae to laryngeal ventricle. Glottis includes the true vocal cord along with anterior and posterior commissure. Subglottis extends from undersurface of true vocal cords to cricoid.

Section 1: Cross-Sectional Anatomy on CT Scan

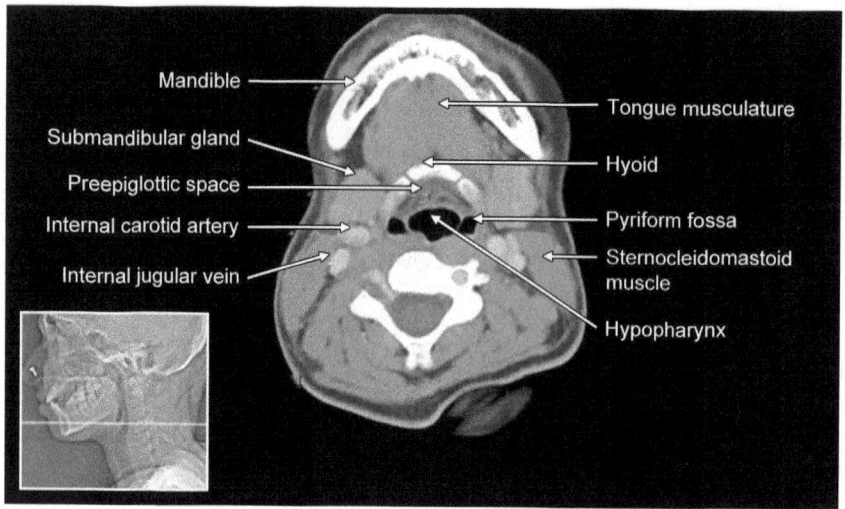

Fig. 5: Axial CT section of neck—level hypopharynx.

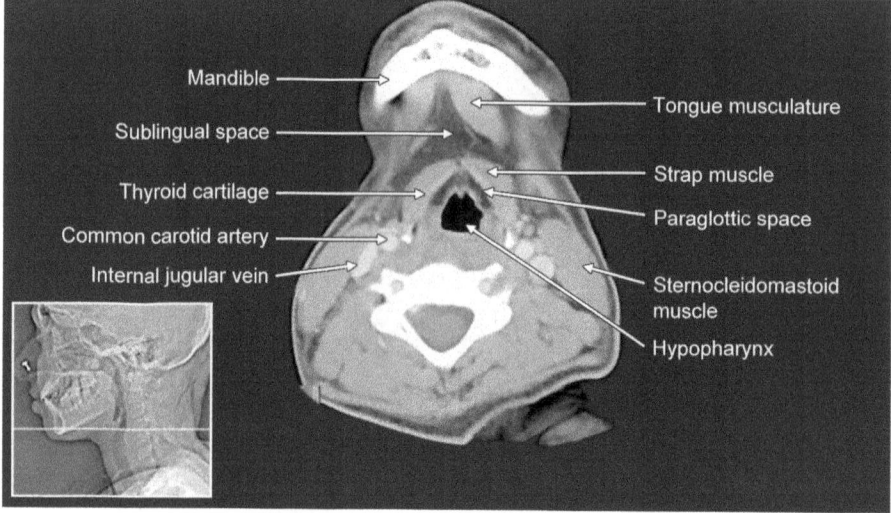

Fig. 6: Axial CT section of neck—level thyroid cartilage.

Deep spaces of suprahyoid portion of neck are:
- Masticator space
- Pharyngeal mucosal space
- Parapharyngeal space
- Retropharyngeal space
- Prevertebral space
- Carotid space
- Parotid space
- Submandibular space

Chapter 5: Face and Neck

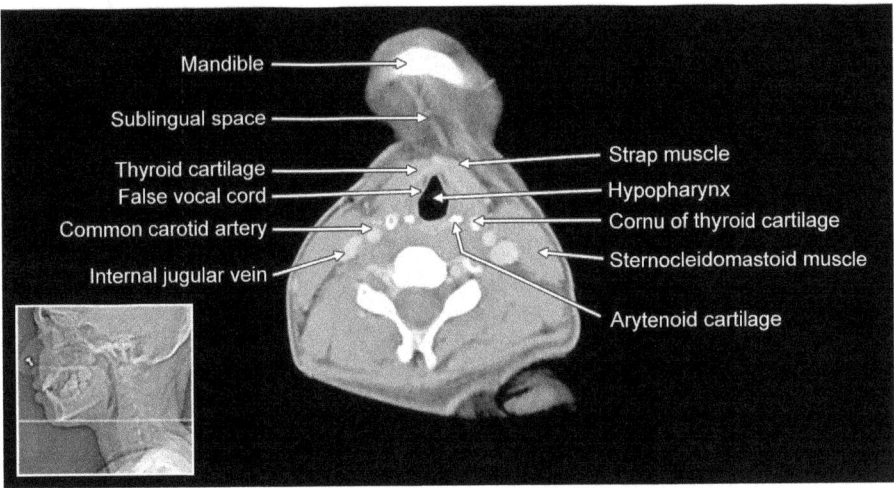

Fig. 7: Axial CT section of neck—level arytenoid cartilage.

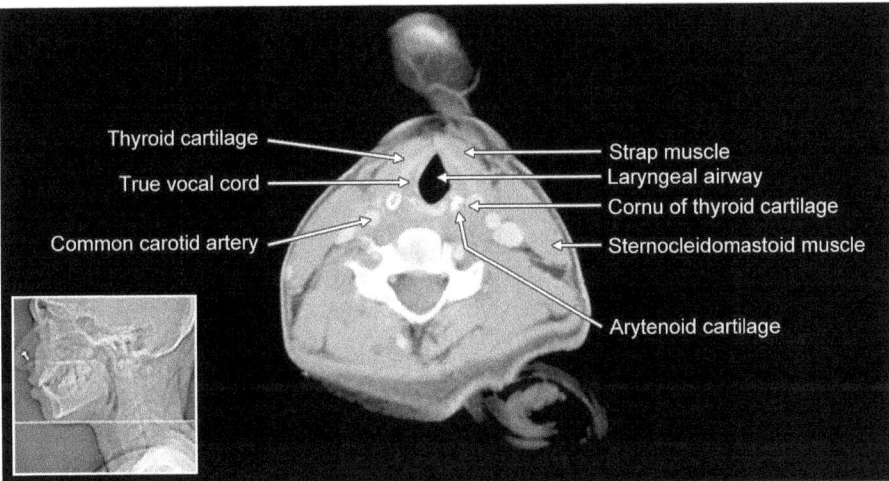

Fig. 8: Axial CT section of neck—level true vocal cords.

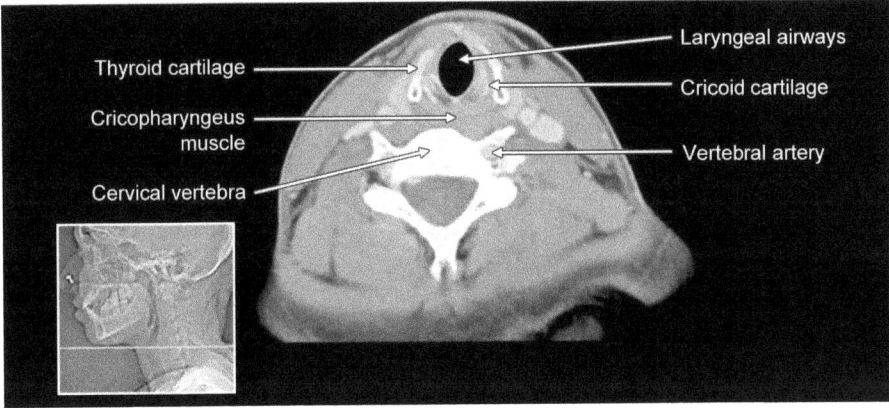

Fig. 9: Axial CT section of neck—level cricoid cartilage.

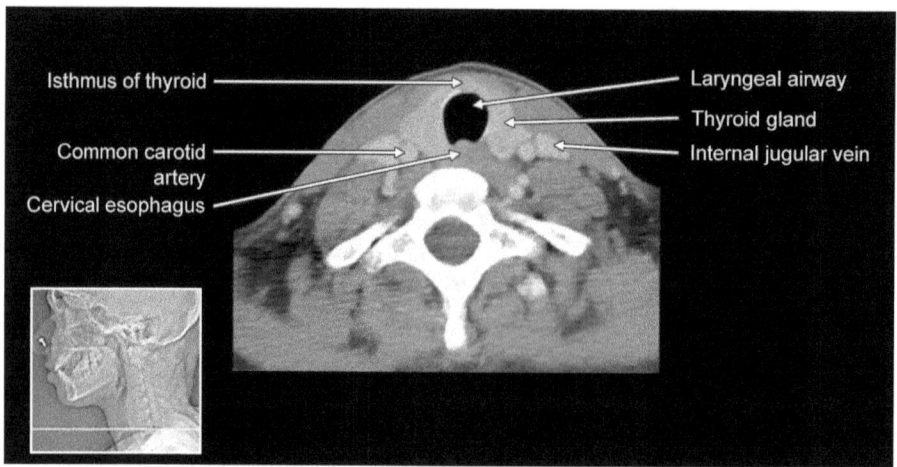

Fig. 10: Axial CT section of neck—level isthmus of thyroid gland.

SALIVARY GLANDS

There are three pairs of salivary glands: Parotids, submandibular and sublingual glands.

Parotid gland is located in the parotid space at the angle of mandible. It has a superficial lobe (which forms the main bulk), deep lobe and an accessory lobe. It is drained by Stensen's duct that opens opposite the upper second molar tooth.

Thyroid gland appears slightly hyperdense on CT scan and has a value of 60–120 HU.

Parathyroid glands are four in number. Two superior parathyroid and two inferior parathyroid glands. Rarely supernumerary parathyroid glands can be seen between 6–12 in number.

CHAPTER 6

Vertebral Column

It is formed by 33 bones called vertebrae which are connected with each other by joints and have a cushion of intervertebral disc in between. A typical vertebra has a body, pedicle anteriorly, transverse process laterally, lamina posterolaterally and spinous process posteriorly. Vertebral column is made of cervical, thoracic, lumbar, sacral and coccygeal vertebrae.
1. Anterior column is formed by anterior longitudinal ligament, anterior annulus fibrosus and anterior part of vertebral body.
2. Middle column is formed by posterior longitudinal ligament, posterior annulus fibrosus and posterior part of vertebral body.
3. Posterior column includes posterior elements and ligaments.

CRANIOVERTEBRAL JUNCTION

Chamberlain line is the line between posterior part of hard palate and posterior margin of foramen magnum. Normally the tip of odontoid process lies at or below this line.

Basilar line is the line along the clivus and it usually falls tangent to posterior aspect of tip of odontoid.

Craniovertebral angle (clivus-canal angle) is angle between basilar line and a line along posterior aspect of odontoid process. If this angle is <150°, cord compression can occur on the ventral aspect.

COVERINGS OF SPINAL CORD

- Periosteum is formed by continuation of outer layer of cerebral dura mater.
- Epidural space is between dura mater and bone and contains epidural veins, lymphatics, fat and connective tissues.
- Dura mater is the continuation of inner layer of cerebral dura mater and ends at second lumbar vertebral level. It sends extensions around spinal nerves and continues with epineurium of peripheral nerves.
- Subarachnoid space extends between arachnoid and pia mater. It contains CSF.
- Pia mater is firmly adherent to spinal cord.

VERTEBRAL CANAL

If the conus medullaris is at or below L3 vertebral level rule out tethering of cord, bony spur or thick filum.
- Axial CT images of occipital condyles/base of skull (**Fig. 1**), C1 vertebra/atlas (**Figs. 2 and 3**), C2 vertebra/axis (**Figs. 4 and 5**).
- Coronal CT images of atlanto-occipital and atlanto-axial junctions (**Fig. 6**).
- Axial CT image of typical cervical vertebra (**Fig. 7**).
- Volume rendered CT images C1-C2 level; axial view (**Fig. 8**), coronal view (**Fig. 9**) and sagittal view (**Fig. 10**).

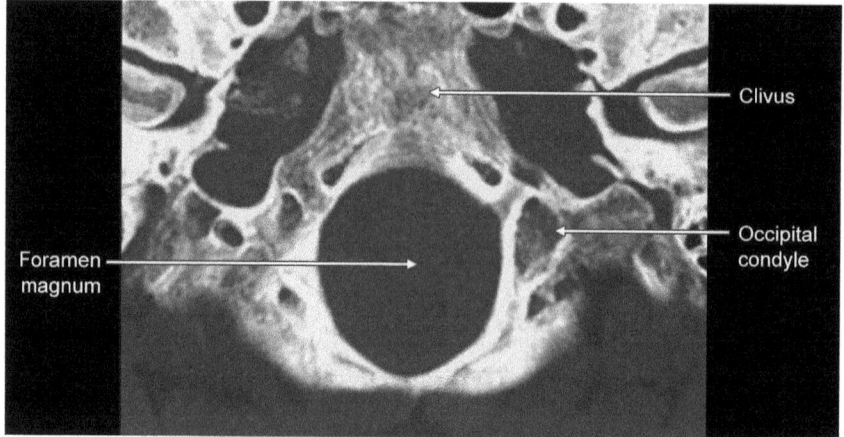

Fig. 1: Occipital condyle.

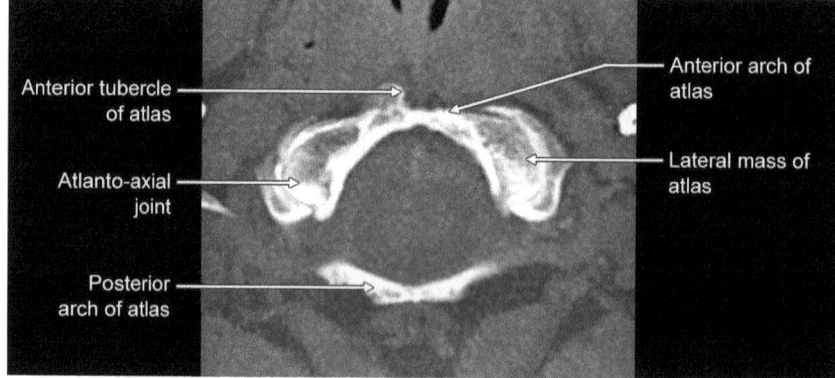

Fig. 2: C1 vertebra (atlas).

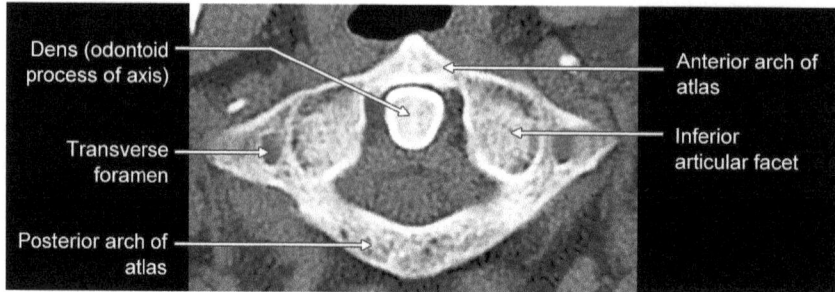

Fig. 3: C1 vertebra.

Chapter 6: Vertebral Column

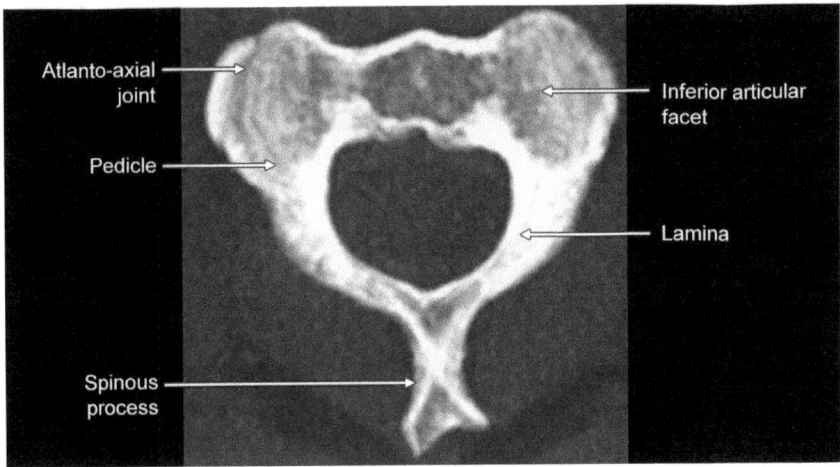

Fig. 4: C2 vertebra (axis).

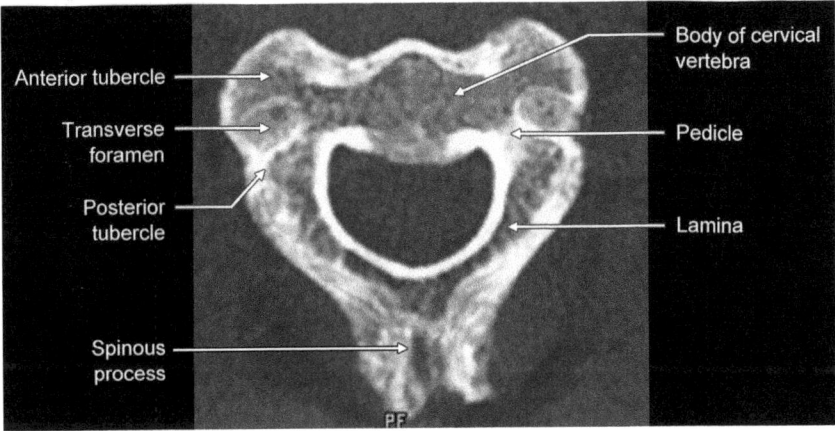

Fig. 5: C2 vertebra.

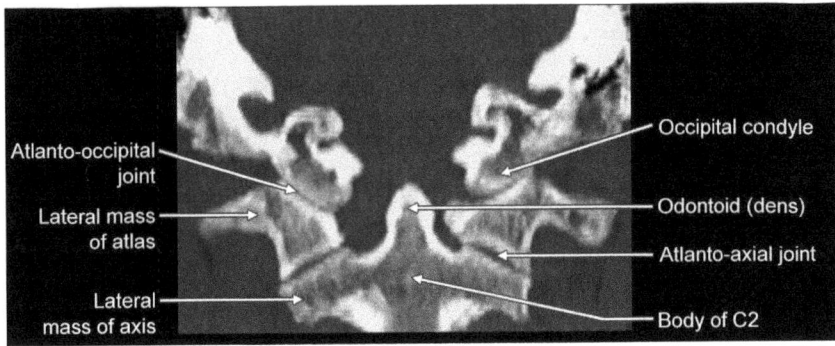

Fig. 6: C1-C2 coronal reconstruction.

Section 1: Cross-Sectional Anatomy on CT Scan

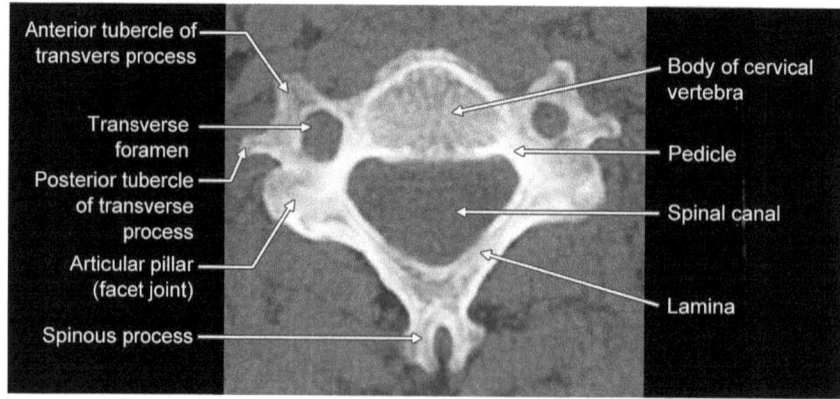

Fig. 7: Typical cervical vertebra (C3-C7).

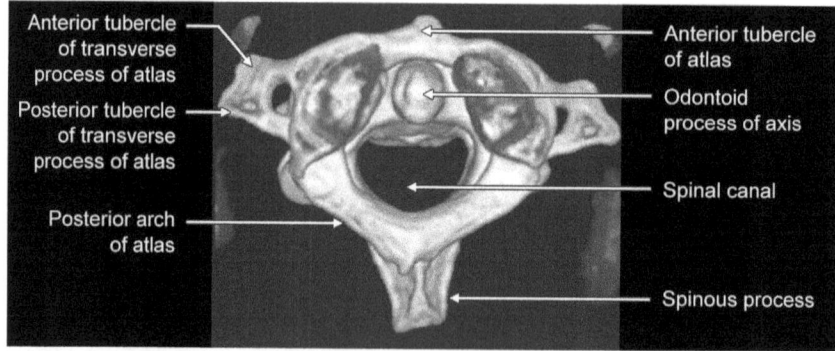

Fig. 8: Axial view (C1-C2 level) volume rendered image.

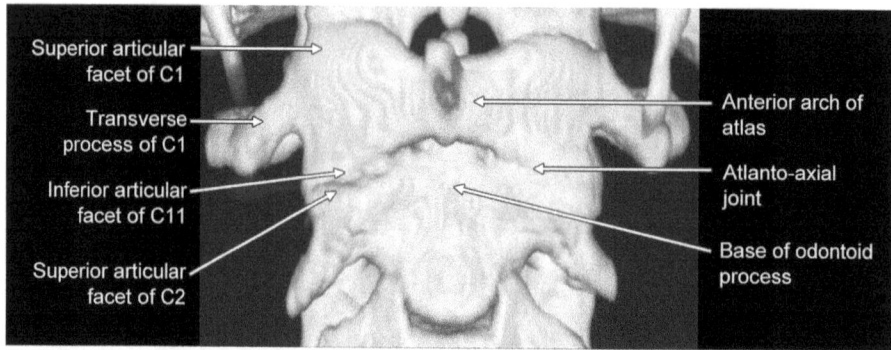

Fig. 9: Coronal view (C1-C2 level) volume rendered image.

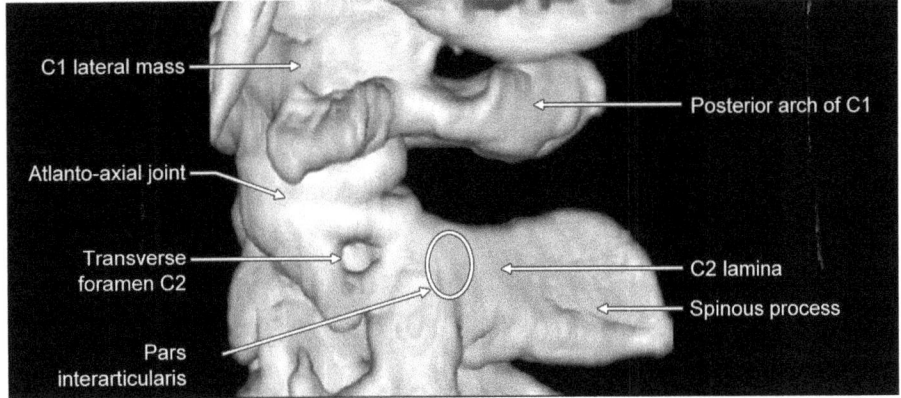

Fig. 10: Sagittal view (C1-C2 level) volume rendered image.

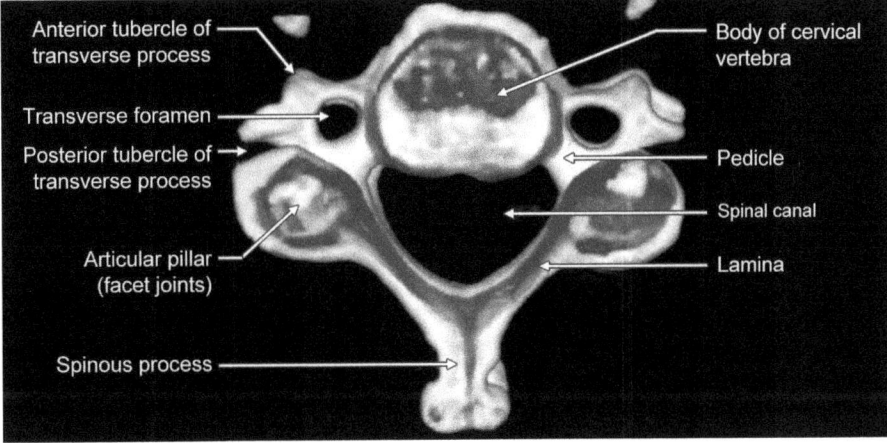

Fig. 11: Axial typical vertebra (C3-C7) volume rendered image.

* Volume rendered CT images of other cervical vertebrae; axial view **(Fig. 11)**, coronal view **(Fig. 12)** and sagittal view **(Fig. 13)**.
* Axial CT image of typical thoracic vertebra **(Fig. 14)**.
* Coronal CT image of thoracolumbar junction **(Fig. 15)**.
* Volume rendered CT images of thoracic spine; coronal view **(Fig. 16)** and sagittal view **(Fig. 17)**.
* Axial CT images of typical lumbar vertebra **(Fig. 18)** and sacroiliac region **(Fig. 19)**.
* Coronal CT image of lumbosacral region **(Fig. 20)**.

Section 1: Cross-Sectional Anatomy on CT Scan

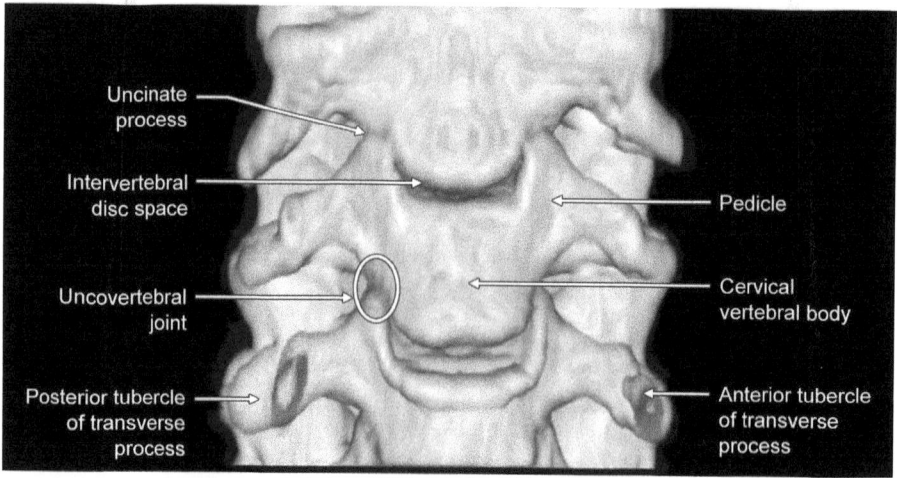

Fig. 12: Coronal view (C2-C4 level) volume rendered image.

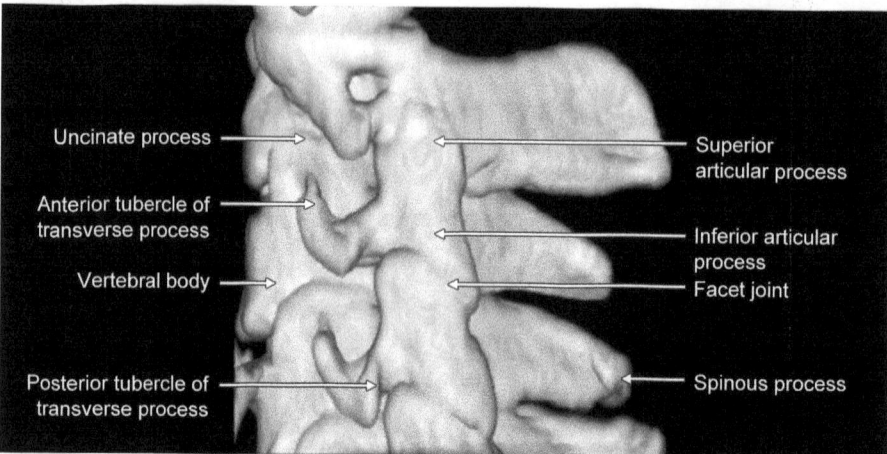

Fig. 13: Sagittal view (C2-C4 level) volume rendered image.

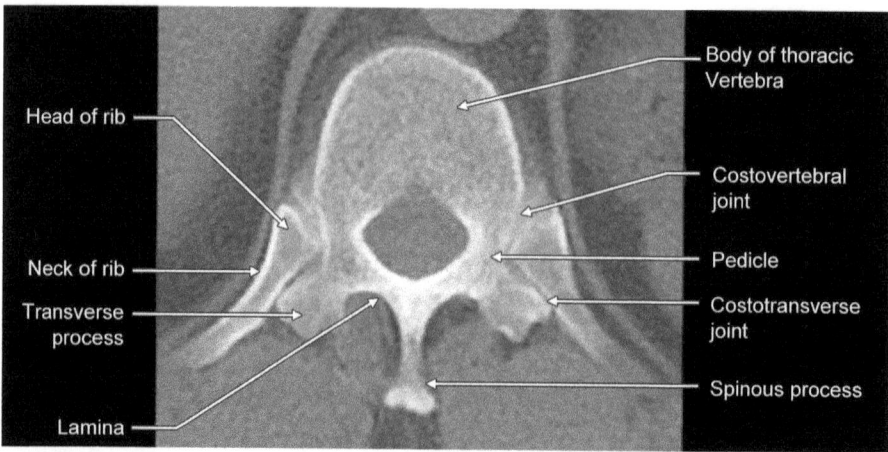

Fig. 14: Typical thoracic vertebra.

Chapter 6: Vertebral Column

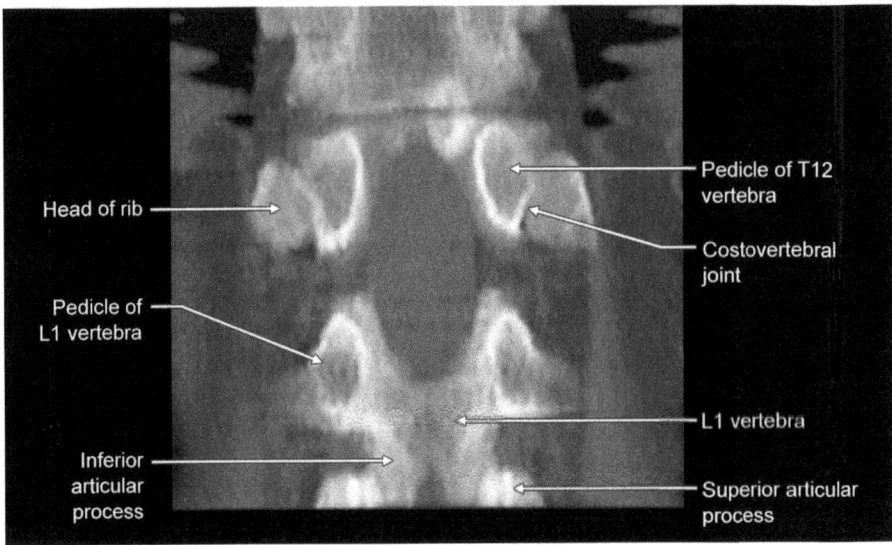

Fig. 15: T12-L1 coronal.

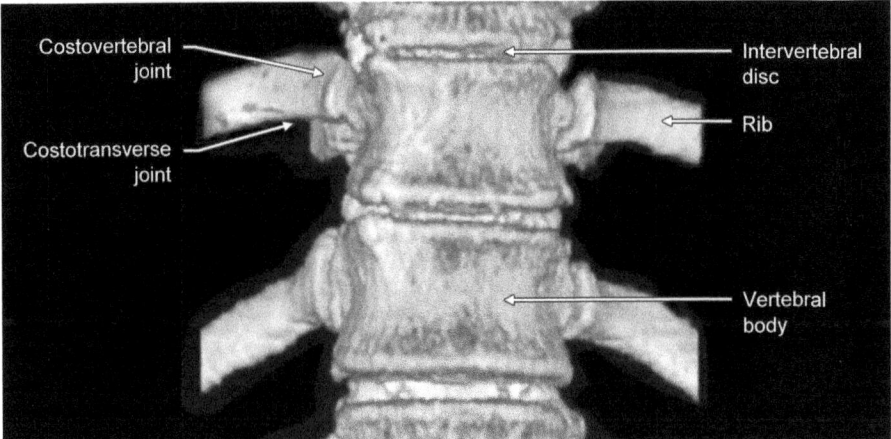

Fig. 16: Coronal view (typical thoracic vertebrae).

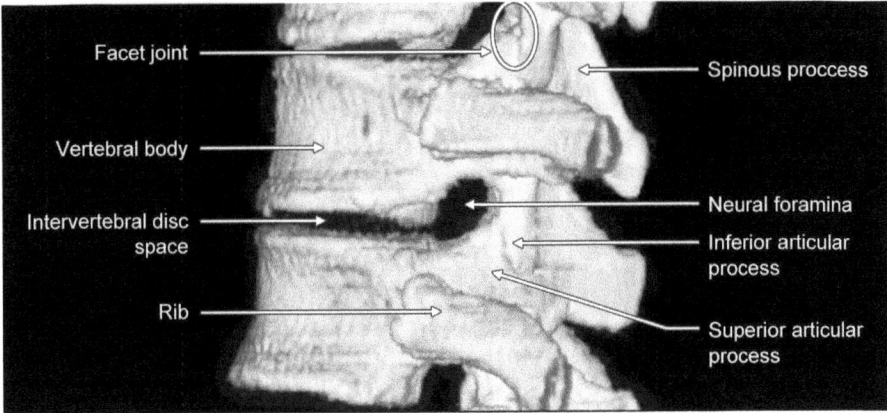

Fig. 17: Sagittal recon showing typical thoracic vertebrae.

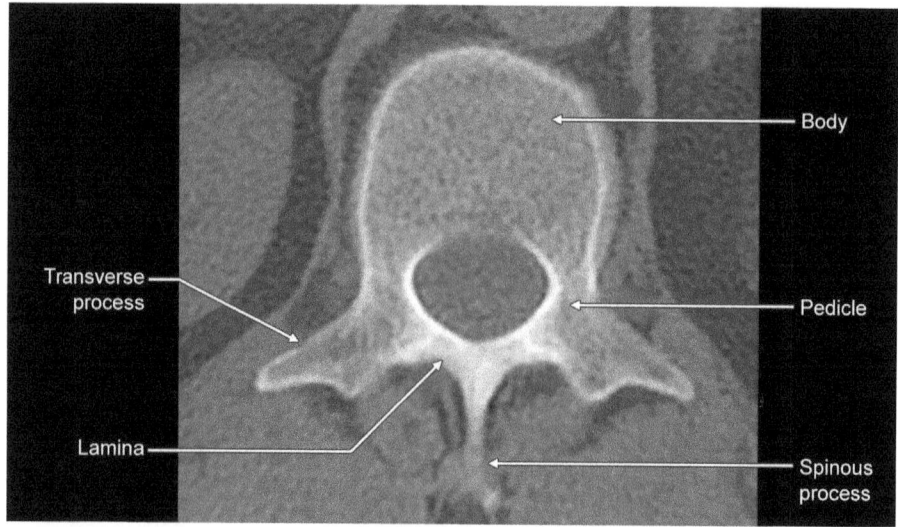
Fig. 18: Typical lumbar vertebra.

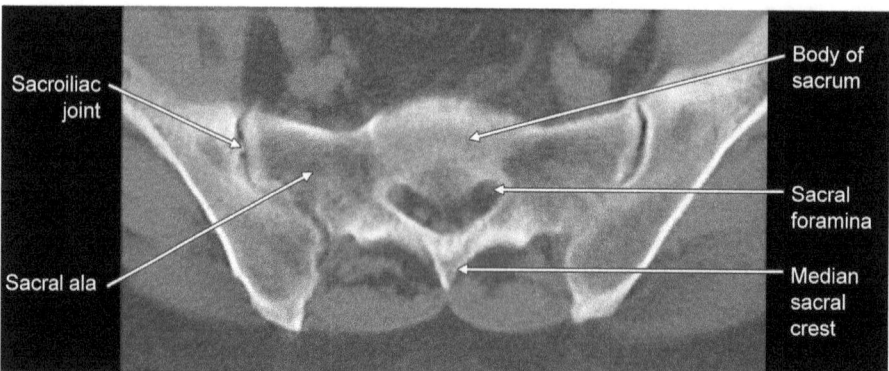
Fig. 19: S1 vertebra and sacroiliac joints.

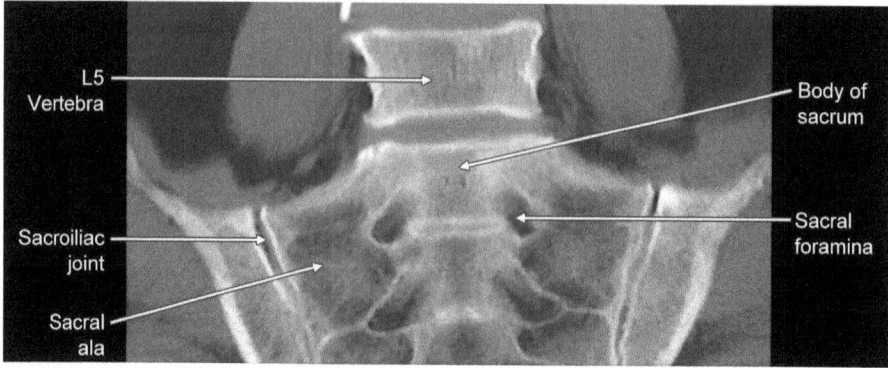
Fig. 20: L5-S1 coronal recon.

CHAPTER 7

Chest and Mediastinum

Embryologically airway starts developing by fifth week of gestational age in the form of lung buds which grow from ventral aspect of primitive foregut. Trachea and esophagus are also separated by fifth week. Hereafter tracheobronchial tree is formed from fifth to fifteenth week. There are 23–25 airway generations from trachea to bronchiole. Bronchus has cartilage in the wall, whereas bronchiole is devoid of cartilage.

Interstitium of lung is divided into axial interstitium, parenchymal interstitial interstitium and peripheral interstitium. Axial interstitium is made of bronchovascular sheaths and lymphatics. Parenchymal interstitium includes interalveolar septum along alveolar walls. Peripheral interstitium includes subpleural connective tissue and interlobular septa which encloses the pulmonary veins and lymphatics.

Pulmonary circulation includes primary pulmonary circulation, bronchial circulation and the anastomosis between the two. Primary pulmonary circulation consists of pulmonary arteries and veins that travel down to subsegmental bronchial level and has a diameter same as that of the accompanying airway. Main pulmonary artery arises from the right ventricle.

Bronchial circulation originates from thoracic aorta and supplies through the intercostal arteries which are two in number for each lung.

SEGMENTAL DIVISION OF LUNGS

Right lung has three lobes:
1. Upper lobe which has an apical, anterior and a posterior segment.
2. Middle lobe has a lateral and a medial segment.
3. Lower lobe has superior segment, medial basal segment, anterior basal segment, lateral basal segment and a posterior basal segment.

Left lung has two lobes:
1. Upper lobe which has an apicoposterior, anterior, superior lingular and an inferior lingular segment.
2. Lower lobe has superior segment, anterior basal segment, lateral basal segment and a posterior basal segment.
   Left lung has no middle lobe.

MEDIASTINUM

Mediastinum is the space between the lungs. It is divided into a superior and an inferior compartment. Superior compartment consists of the thoracic inlet. Inferior compartment has anterior, middle and posterior subcompartments. Retrosternal region is included in the anterior compartment, heart lies in the middle compartment and descending aorta with esophagus and paraspinal region is located in the posterior mediastinal compartment. Thymus is located in the anterior part of superior as well as inferior compartment of mediastinum.

Window Settings for Chest and Mediastinum

Window settings for evaluating the lung are window-width 1500 HU and window-level (-)600 HU. Window settings for evaluating the mediastinum are window-width 350 HU and window-level 40 HU.

Window Level

The window level (WL), often also referred to as window center, is the midpoint of the range of the CT numbers displayed. When the window level is decreased the CT image will be brighter and vice versa.

Window Width

The window width selects the range of Hounsfield units for a particular image, and the window level determines the center of Hounsfield units in this range. In general, the window level is set at roughly the same level as the Hounsfield value of the tissue of interest.

Lung Window

A lung window is used to view lung parenchyma **(Figs. 1 to 12)**. Lung parenchyma (–500 HU) would be within range, appearing gray. Air pockets (–1000 HU) around the lung, such as pneumothorax or bullae, would appear black, thus allowing clear differentiation.

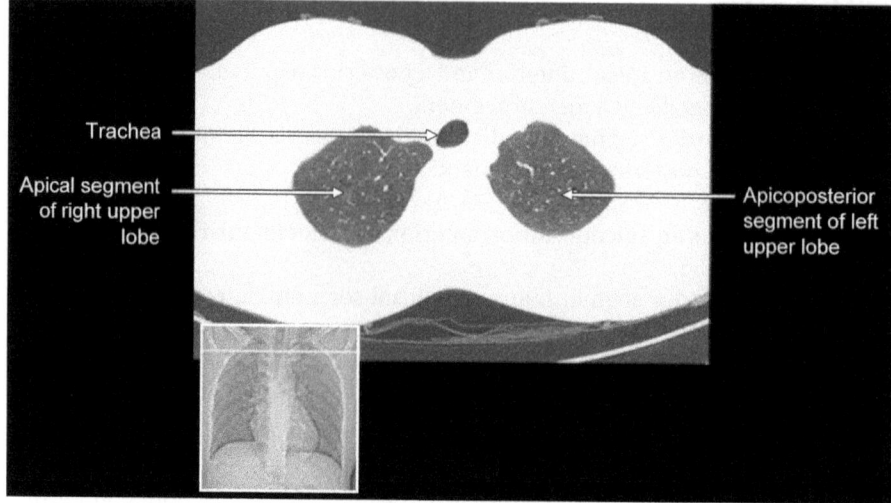

Fig. 1: Axial CT section chest (lung window) apices.

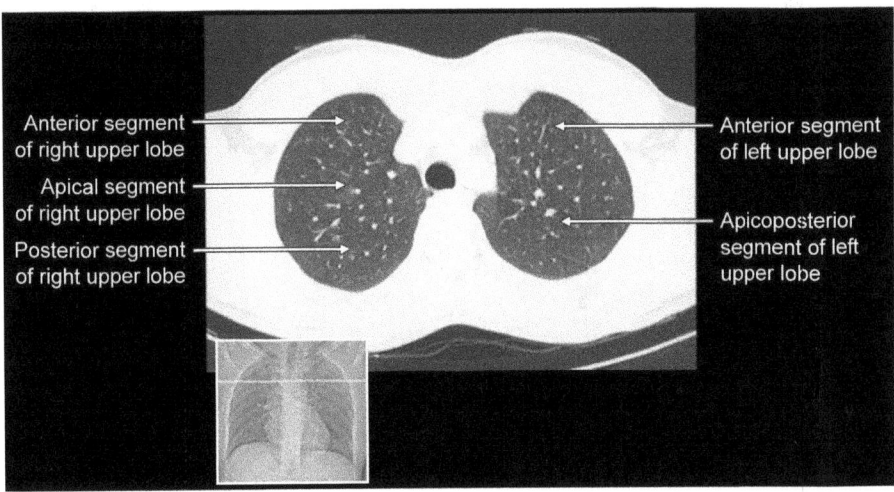

Fig. 2: Axial CT section chest (lung window)—anterior segment.

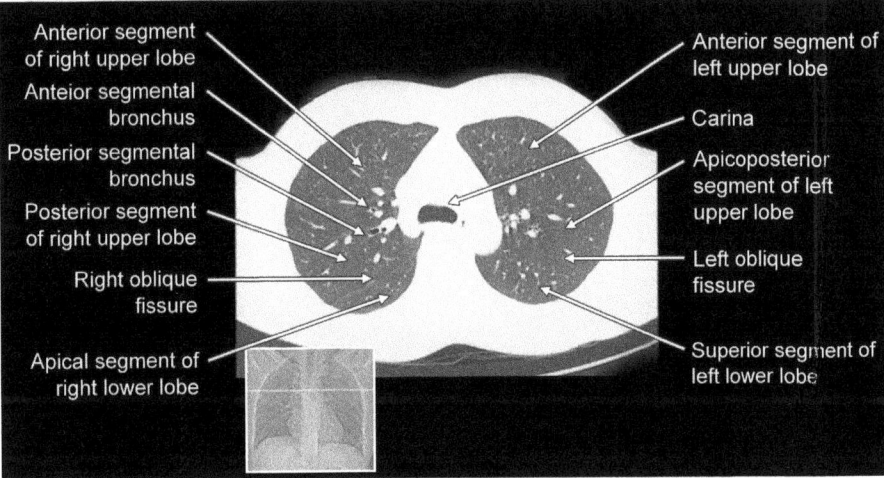

Fig. 3: Axial CT section chest (lung window) at the level of carina.

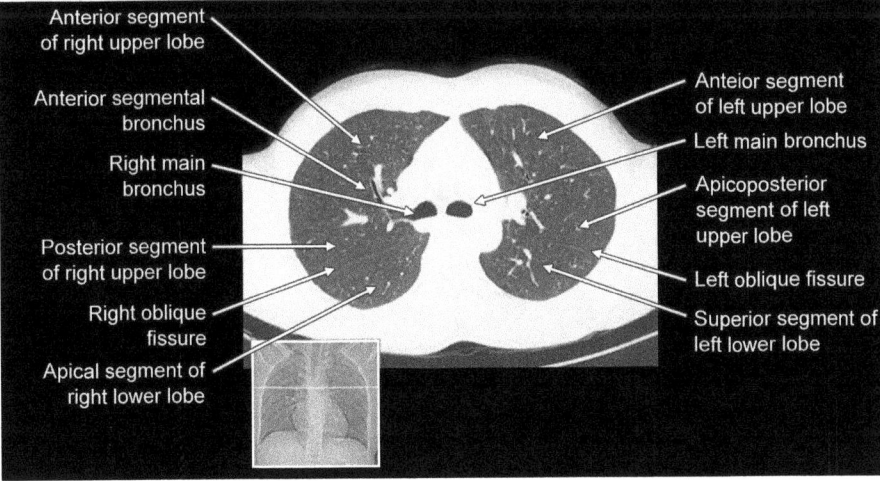

Fig. 4: Axial CT section chest (lung window) at the level of bronchi.

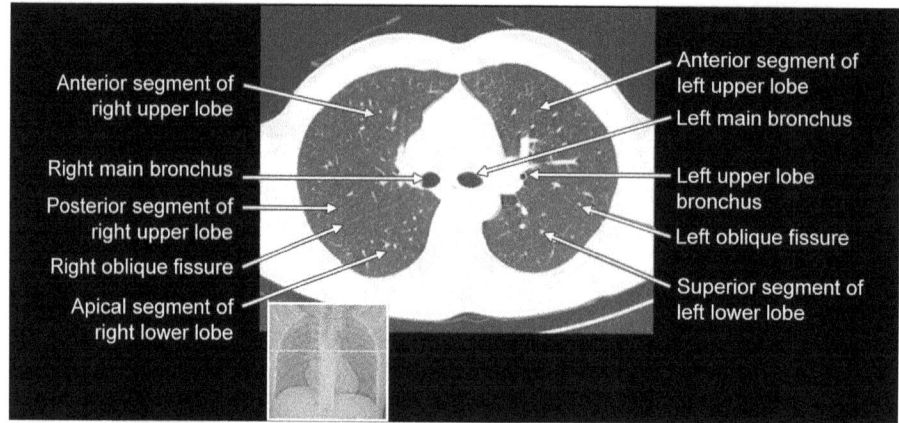

Fig. 5: Axial CT section chest (lung window) showing anterior segment.

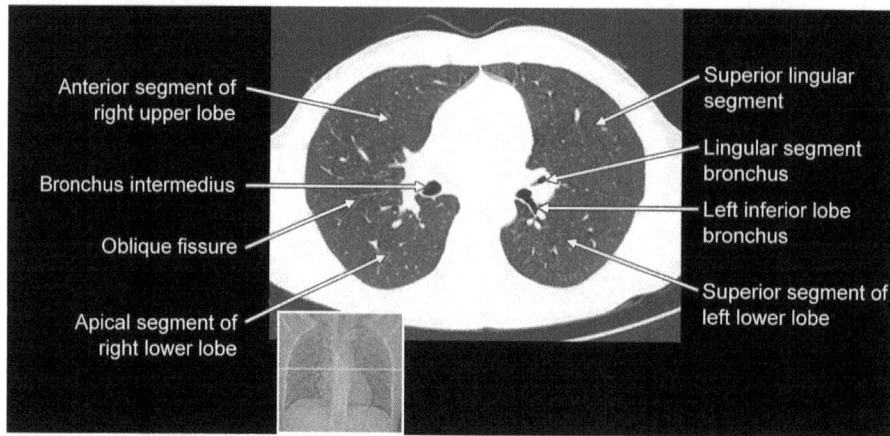

Fig. 6: Axial CT section chest (lung window) at the level of hilum.

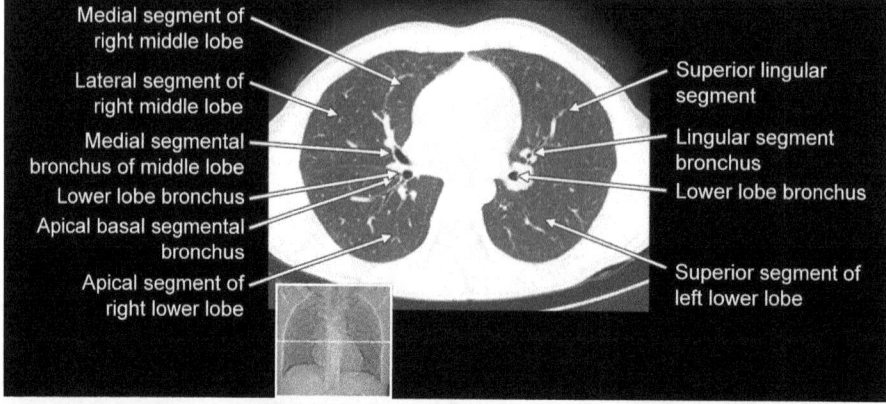

Fig. 7: Axial CT section chest (lung window) at the level of lingular segments and middle lobes.

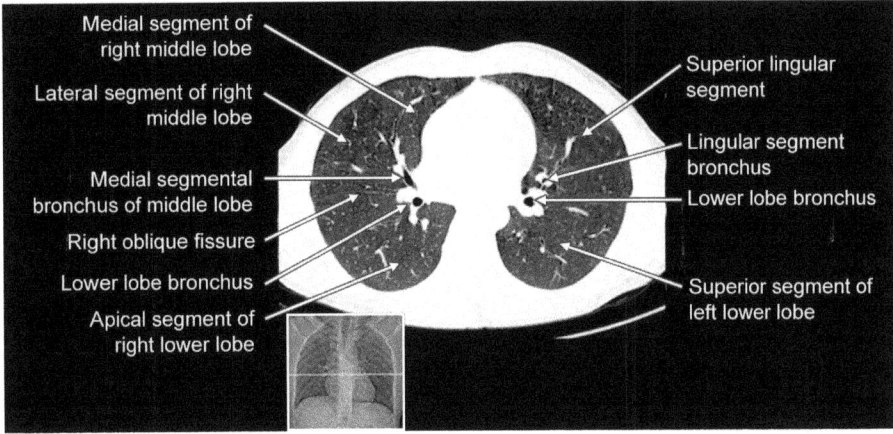

Fig. 8: Axial CT section chest (lung window) at the level of apical segments of lower lobe.

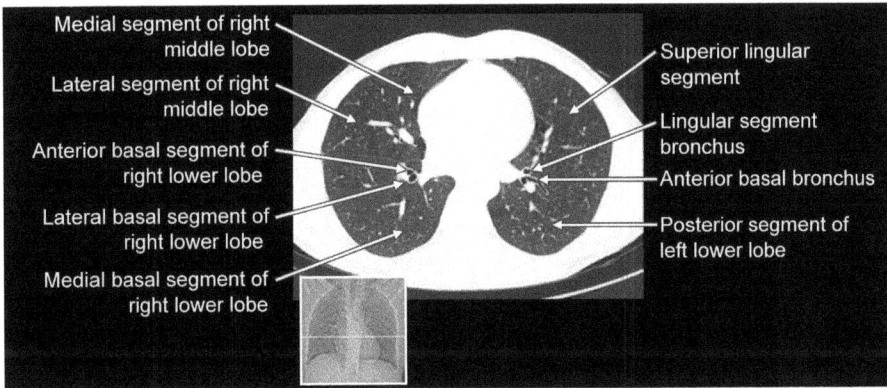

Fig. 9: Axial CT section chest (lung window) showing lingual, middle and lower lobes.

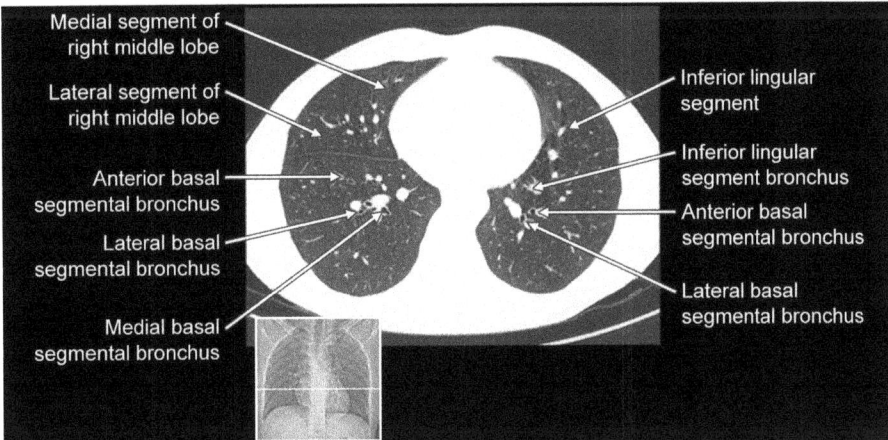

Fig. 10: Axial CT section chest (lung window) showing middle and lower lobes.

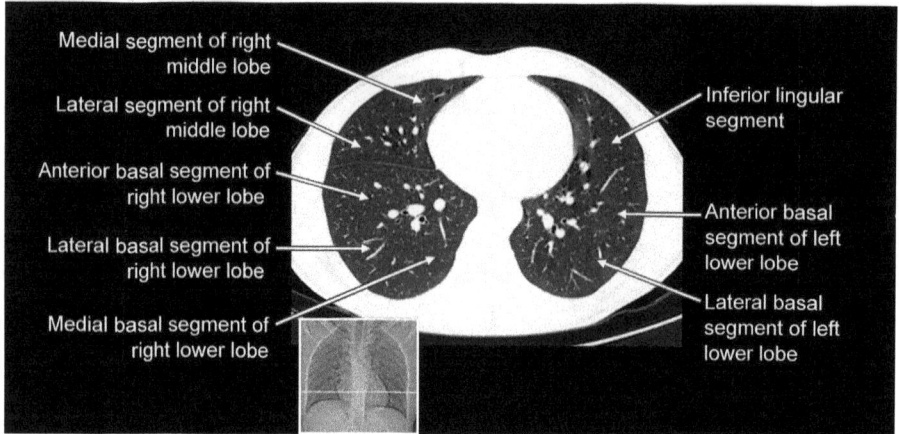

Fig. 11: Axial CT section chest (lung window) showing lower lobes.

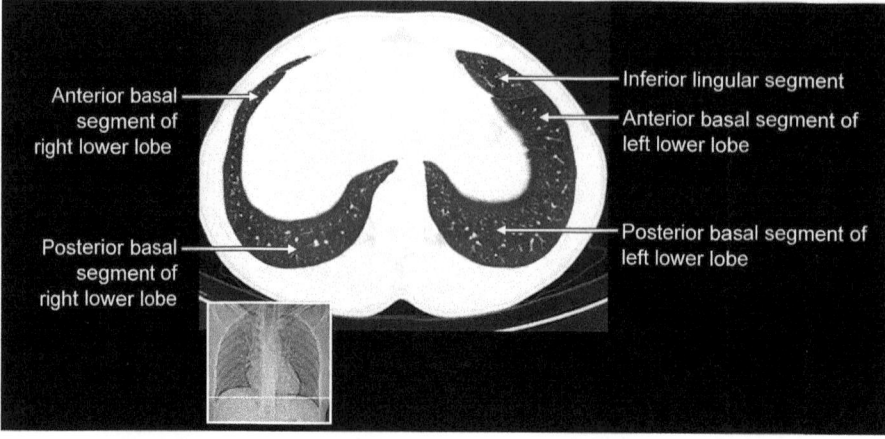

Fig. 12: Axial CT section chest (lung window) at the level of diaphragm.

Mediastinal Window

In the mediastinal window the lungs are overexposed and simply appear black **(Figs. 13 to 20)**. This algorithm is used to assess chest wall and mediastinal structures, usually with intravenous contrast so that vascular structures in the mediastinum can be distinguished from enlarged lymph nodes or other masses.

CT MEDIASTINUM

Normal Anatomy

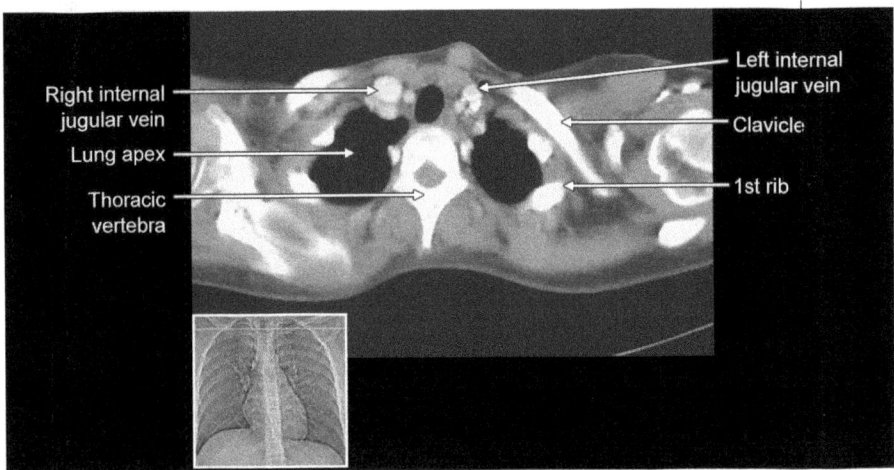

Fig. 13: Axial CT section of chest showing lung apex in mediastinal window at the level of internal jugular vein.

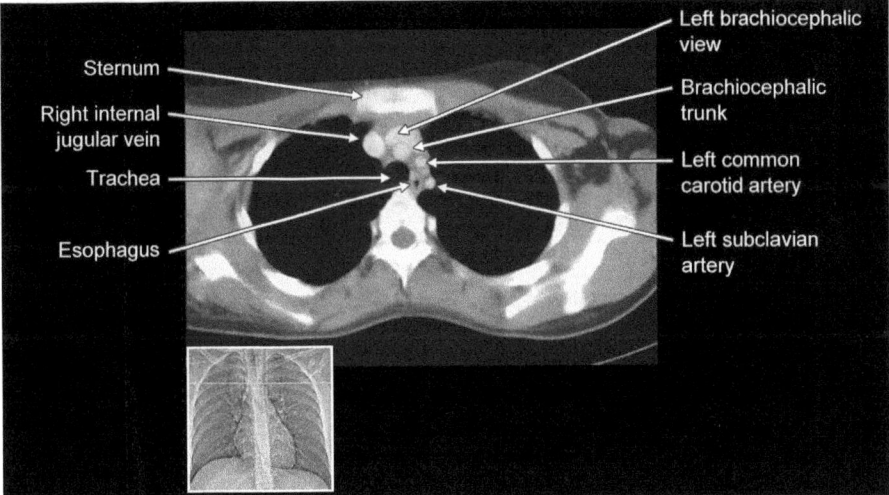

Fig. 14: Axial CT section of chest in mediastinal window at the level of branches of arch of aorta.

Section 1: Cross-Sectional Anatomy on CT Scan

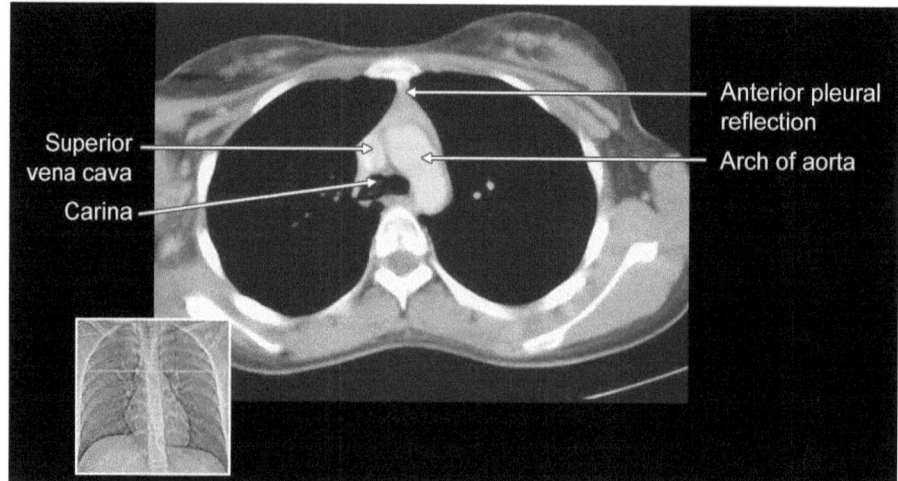

Fig. 15: Axial CT section of chest in mediastinal window at the level of arch of aorta.

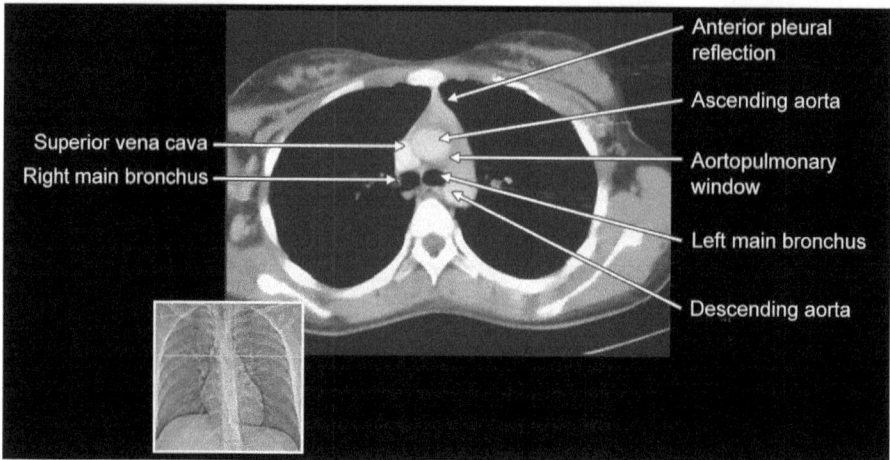

Fig. 16: Axial CT section of chest in mediastinal window at the level of ascending and descending thoracic aorta.

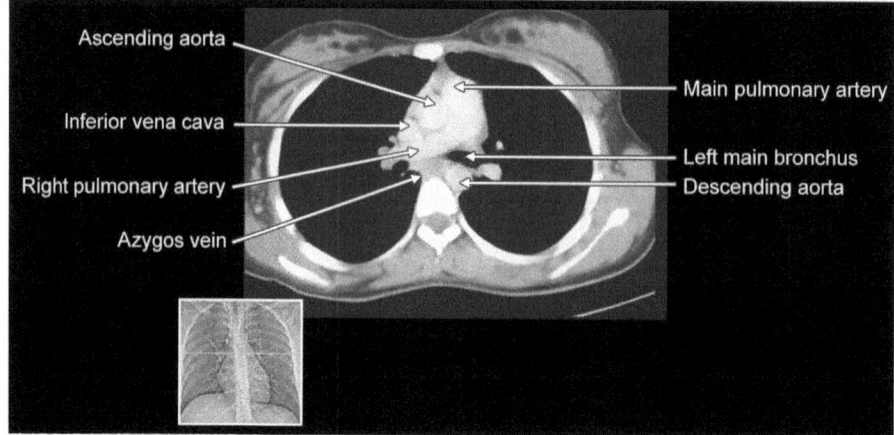

Fig. 17: Axial CT section of chest in mediastinal window at the level of main pulmonary artery.

Chapter 7: Chest and Mediastinum

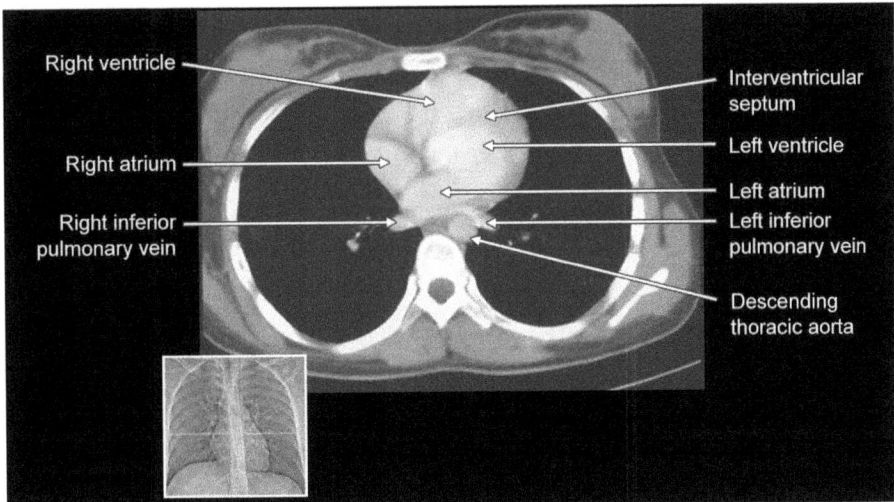

Fig. 18: Axial CT section of chest in mediastinal window showing chambers of heart.

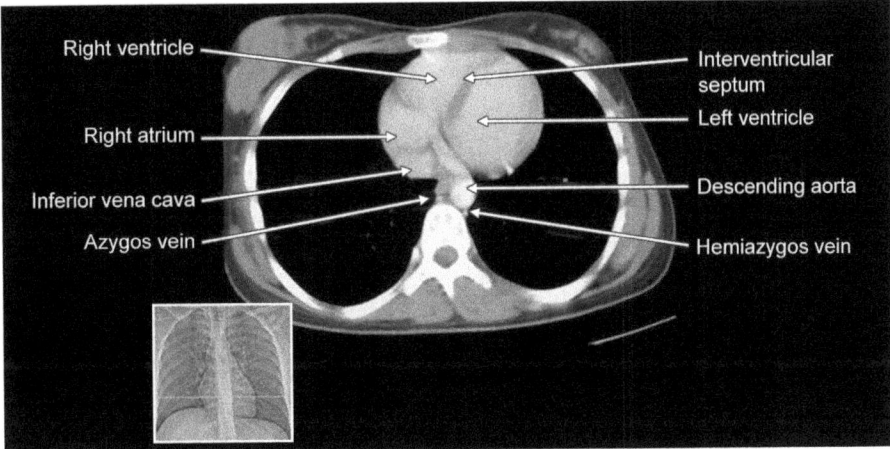

Fig. 19: Axial CT section of chest in mediastinal window showing heart chambers and azygos and hemiazygos veins.

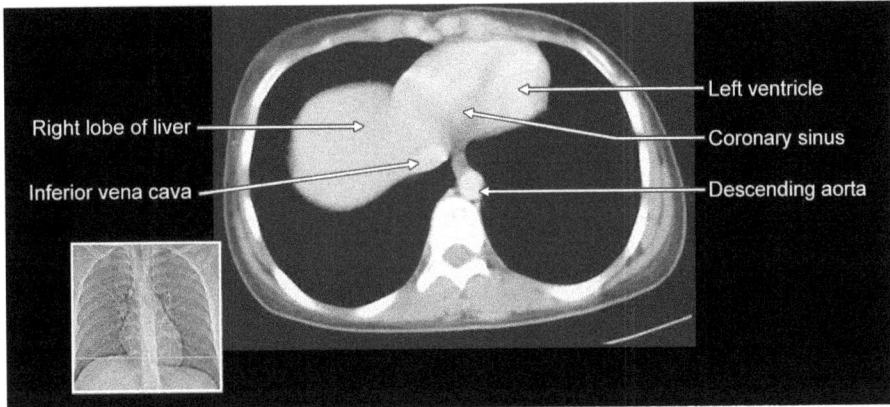

Fig. 20: Axial CT section of chest in mediastinal window at the level of liver.

CHAPTER 8

Heart

CT NORMAL CORONARY ANGIOGRAPHY

Heart imaging methods such as cardiac CT are allowing physicians to take a closer look at the heart and great vessels with little risk to the patient.

A traditional CT scan is an X-ray procedure which combines many X-ray images with the aid of a computer to generate cross-sectional views of the body. Cardiac CT uses advanced CT technology with or without intravenous iodine-based contrast to visualize cardiac anatomy including the coronary arteries and great arteries and veins. With multidetector scanning, it is possible to acquire high-resolution three-dimensional images of the heart and great vessels.

Cardiac CT is especially useful in evaluating the myocardium, coronary arteries, pulmonary veins, thoracic aorta, pericardium, and cardiac masses, such as thrombus of the left atrial appendage (LAA).

Coronary Arteries

The four main coronary arteries evaluated by CT are the right coronary artery (RCA), the left main coronary artery (LCA), the left anterior descending (LAD) artery, and the left circumflex (LCx) artery **(Figs. 1 to 7)**.

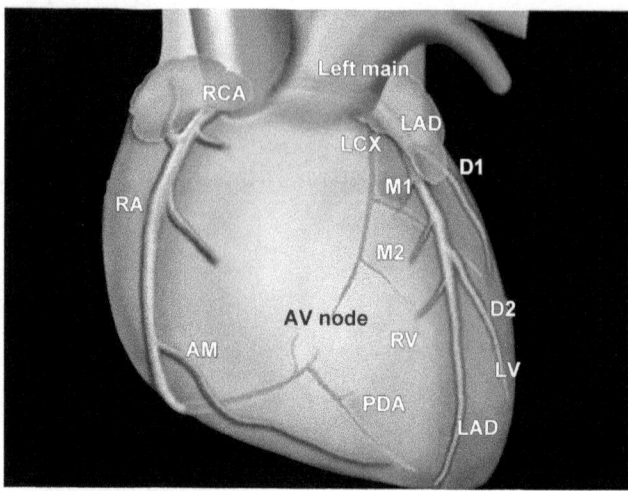

Fig. 1: Heart showing AV node and other coronary arteries.

Chapter 8: Heart

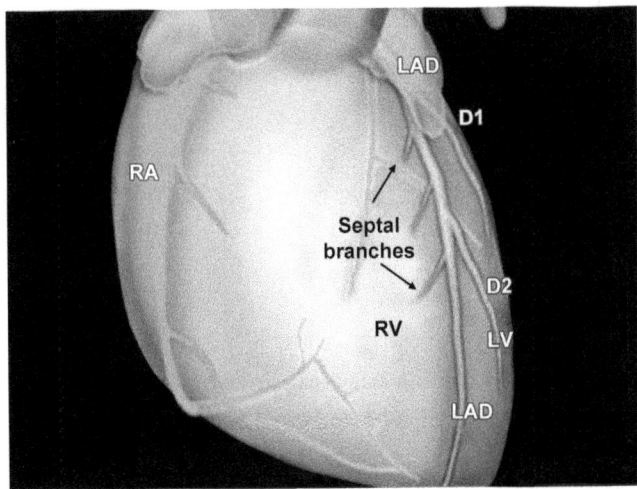

Fig. 2: Heart showing both coronary arteries.

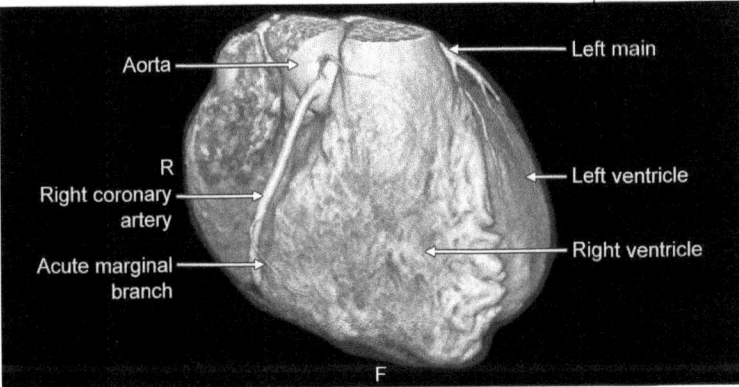

Fig. 3: Heart in coronal plane.

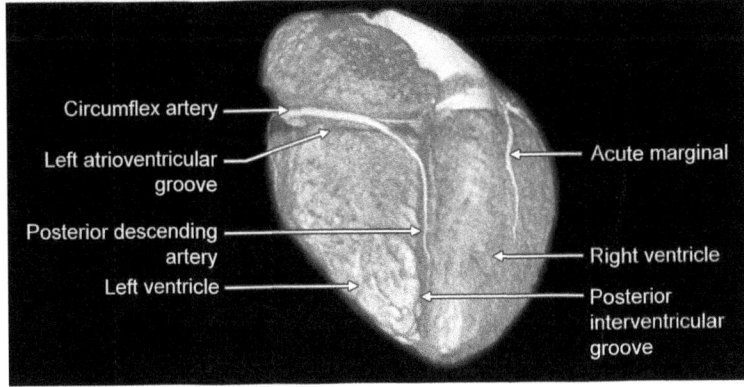

Fig. 4: Posterior oblique coronal plane.

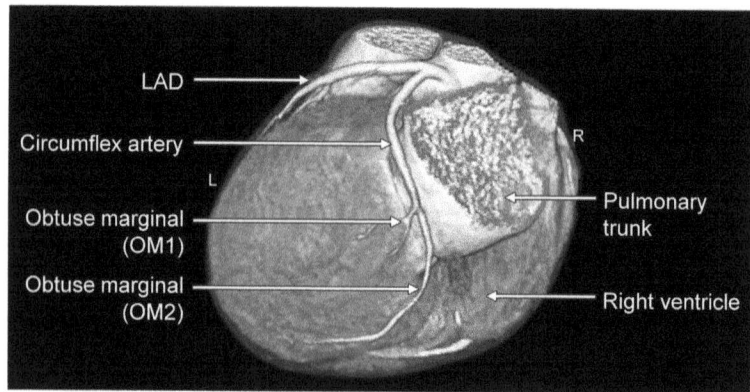

Fig. 5: Coronal plane [maximum intensity projection (MIP) image].

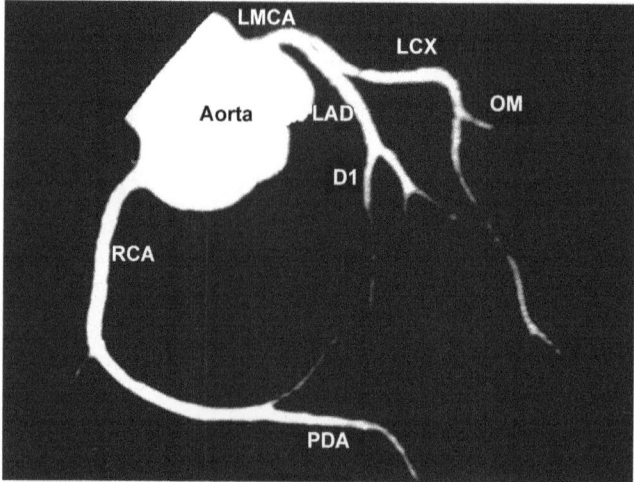

Fig. 6: Axial plane (MIP image).

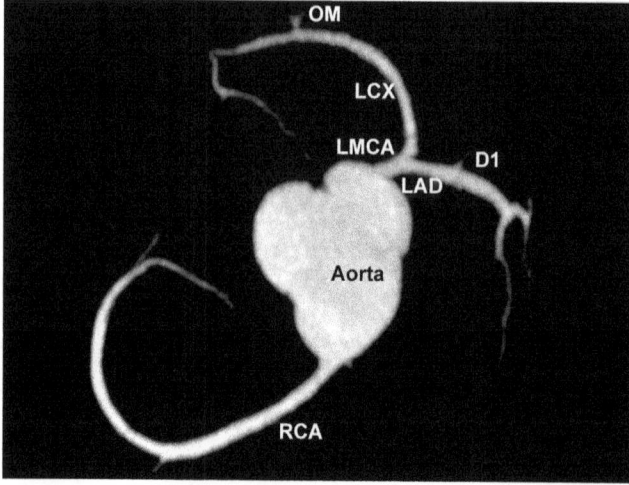

Fig. 7: Oblique coronal plane.

Dominant Coronary Artery

Whichever artery crosses the crux of the heart and gives off the posterior descending branches is considered to be the dominant coronary artery.

In approximately 85% of individuals, the RCA crosses the posterior interventricular groove and gives rise to the posterior descending branches (right dominance); in 7–8%, the LCx artery crosses the interventricular groove and gives rise to branches to the posterior right ventricular surface (left dominance); and in the remaining 7–8%, the inferior interventricular septum is perfused by branches from both the distal RCA and the distal LCx artery (co-dominance).

Right Coronary Artery: The RCA arises from the anterior right coronary sinus somewhat inferior to the origin of the LCA. The RCA passes to the right of and posterior to the pulmonary artery and then downward in the right atrioventricular groove toward the posterior interventricular septum.

In more than 50% of individuals, the first branch of the RCA is the conus artery, unless it (the RCA) has a separate origin directly from the right coronary sinus.

The second branches usually consist of the sinoatrial node/nodal artery and several anterior branches that supply the free wall of the right ventricle.

The branch to the right ventricle at the junction of the middle and distal RCA is called the acute marginal branch.

The distal RCA divides into posterior descending artery (PDA) and posterior left ventricular branches (PLV) in a right dominant anatomy.

Left Coronary Artery: The LCA arises from the left posterior coronary sinus and is 5-10 mm long. The LCA passes to the left of base of ascending aorta and posterior to the pulmonary trunk and bifurcates into the LAD and LCx arteries. Occasionally, the LCA trifurcates into the LAD and LCx arteries and the ramus intermedius. The ramus intermedius has a course similar to that of the first diagonal branch of the LAD artery to the anterior left ventricle.

The LAD artery passes to the left of the pulmonary trunk and turns anteriorly to course in the anterior interventricular groove toward the apex. It provides the diagonal branches (D1 and D2) to the anterior free wall of the left ventricle and the septal branches to the anterior interventricular septum.

The LCx courses in the left atrioventricular groove and gives off obtuse marginal (OM) branches to the lateral left ventricle.

In a left dominant or codominant anatomy, the LCx artery gives rise to the PDA or posterior left ventricular branches.

CHAPTER 9

Abdomen and Pelvis

LIVER

Functional segmental anatomy of liver is based on distribution of three hepatic veins. Middle hepatic vein divides the liver into right and left lobes. Left hepatic vein divides the left lobe into medial and lateral parts. Right hepatic vein divides the right lobe into the anterior and posterior parts. An imaginary transverse line through the right and left portal vein divides these parts into anterior and posterior segments which are numbered counterclockwise from the inferior vena cava (IVC).

The Couinaud classification of liver anatomy divides the liver into eight functionally independent segments (**Figs. 1 to 6**). Each segment has its own vascular inflow, outflow and biliary drainage. In the center of each segment there is a branch of the portal vein, hepatic artery and bile duct. The numbering of the segments is in a clockwise manner.

Segment 1 (caudate lobe) is located posteriorly and extends between fissure of the ligamentum venosum anteriorly and the IVC posteriorly.

The longitudinal plane of the right hepatic vein divides segment 8 from segment 7 in the superior portion of the liver and in the inferior portion of the liver segment 5 from segment 6.

The longitudinal plane of the middle hepatic vein through the gallbladder fossa separates segment 4a from segment 8 in the superior liver and segment 4b from segment 5 in the inferior liver.

The longitudinal plane of the left hepatic vein and fissure of the ligamentum teres separates segment 4a from segment 2 in the superior liver and segment 4b from segment 3 in the inferior liver.

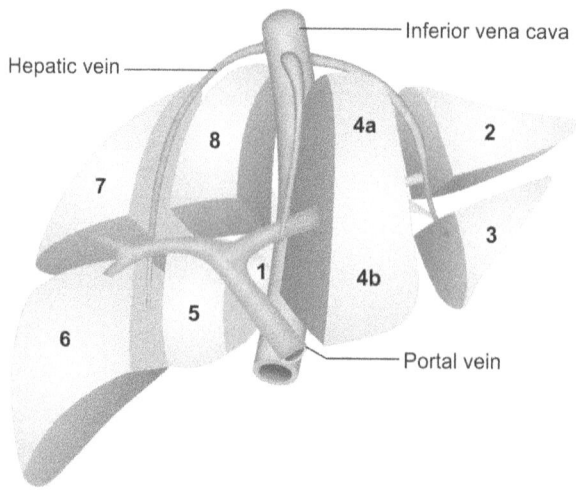

Fig. 1: Liver segments shown diagrammatically (Couinaud classification).

Chapter 9: Abdomen and Pelvis

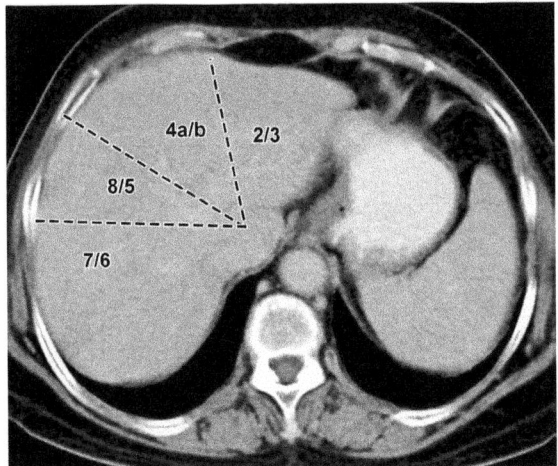

Fig. 2: Liver segments 2 to 8 on CT abdomen.

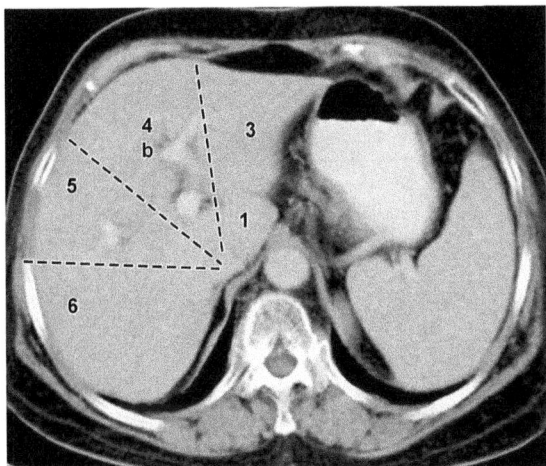

Fig. 3: Liver segments 1, 3 and 6 on CT abdomen.

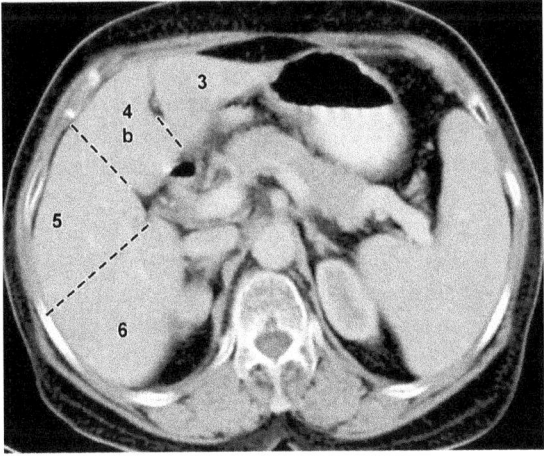

Fig. 4: Axial CT section of abdomen showing liver segments 3, 4b, 5 and 6.

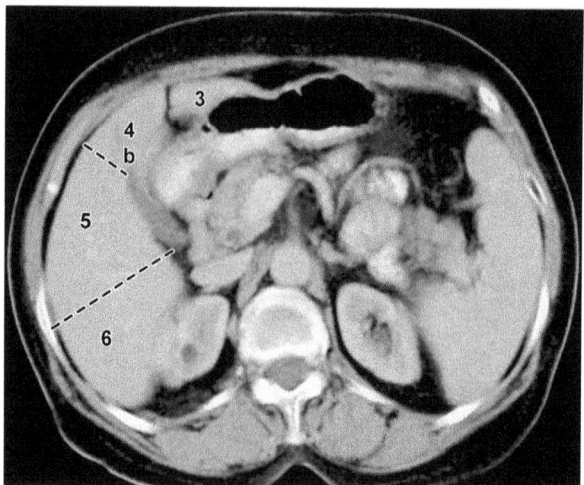

Fig. 5: Axial CT section of abdomen showing liver segments 3 to 6.

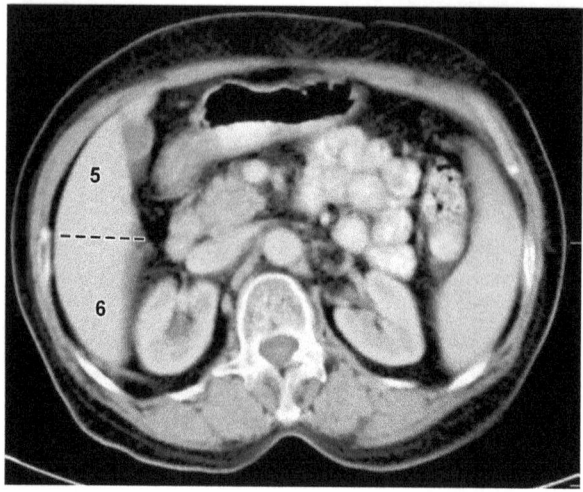

Fig. 6: Axial CT section of abdomen showing liver segments 5 and 6.

The axial plane of the left portal vein separates segment 4a superiorly from segment 4b inferiorly and segment 2 superiorly from segment 3 inferiorly in the left lobe.

The axial plane of the right portal vein separates segment 8 and segment 7 superiorly from segment 5 and segment 6 inferiorly in the right lobe.

Normal liver has a precontrast attenuation value of 45-65 Hounsfield unit (HU) and maximum enhancement occurs at 50-60 seconds after administration of contrast. Normal liver has a size upto 13 cm in craniocaudal extend in adults. Normal portal vein is 10-13 mm in diameter in adults.

GALLBLADDER

Normal gallbladder is upto 10 cm long and 4 cm wide **(Fig. 11)**. It has a normal wall thickness upto 3 mm. Gallbladder may have septae. Bifid appearance is due to longitudinal septum.

Phrygian cap gallbladder is due to kink or septum at the neck. Ectopic gallbladder can be seen beneath the left lobe of liver or even in retrohepatic location. Floating gallbladder can result from loose peritoneal attachments.

Normal cystic duct is 2 cm long and 2 mm wide. Maximum diameter of normal common bile duct in an adult is 2–5 mm. Postcholecystectomy it can be upto 7 mm. Normal width increases by 1 mm per decade in elderly over 60 years of age.

PANCREAS

It develops during the fourth week of gestation as the second endodermal diverticulum from foregut. The dorsal diverticulum forms the dorsal pancreas. Ventral diverticulum forms the ventral pancreas as well as the liver, gallbladder and bile ducts.

The main pancreatic duct is known as the duct of Wirsung. The angle between the pancreatic duct and common bile duct at their joining point is between 5 to 30°. These ducts open into second part of duodenum through the ampulla of Vater which has a sphincter called the sphincter of Oddi.

The entire length of pancreas is 10–15 cm (**Figs. 10 to 13**). Pancreatic tail is upto 1.6 cm thick; body is upto 1.1 cm thick and the head ranges from 1 to 2 cm in thickness.

Annular pancreas is a congenital anomaly in which the duodenum is enclosed on all sides by pancreas as a result of abnormal migration of ventral pancreas.

SPLEEN

Spleen is formed during fifth week of gestational age from mesenchymal cells between layers of dorsal mesogastrium. Accessory spleen can be seen in 10-30 % of patients. Spleen can even be attached to left testis or ovary as there is a close relationship between the left gonadal anlage and the splenic precursor mesenchymal cells (splenogonadal fusion). It has a weight upto 200 gm and a length of 11 cm. The CT value of spleen is 5 HU less than the liver (**Figs. 7 to 11**).

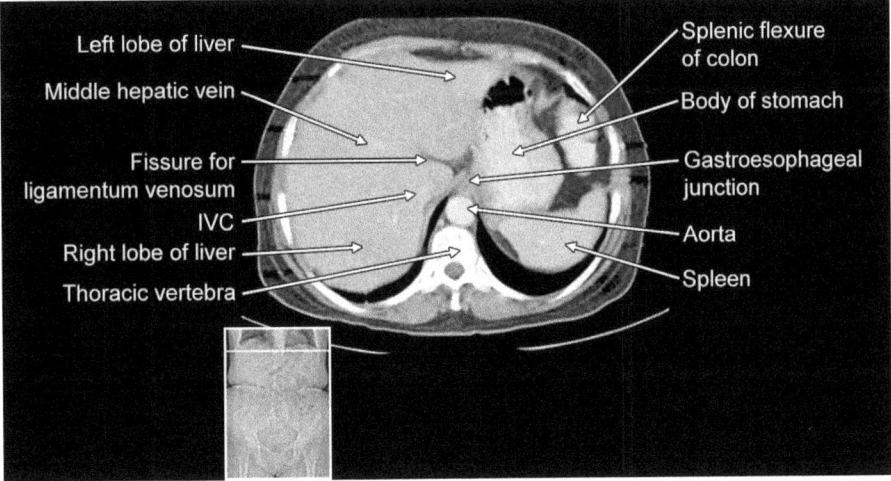

Fig. 7: Axial CT section of abdomen at the level of liver, stomach and spleen.

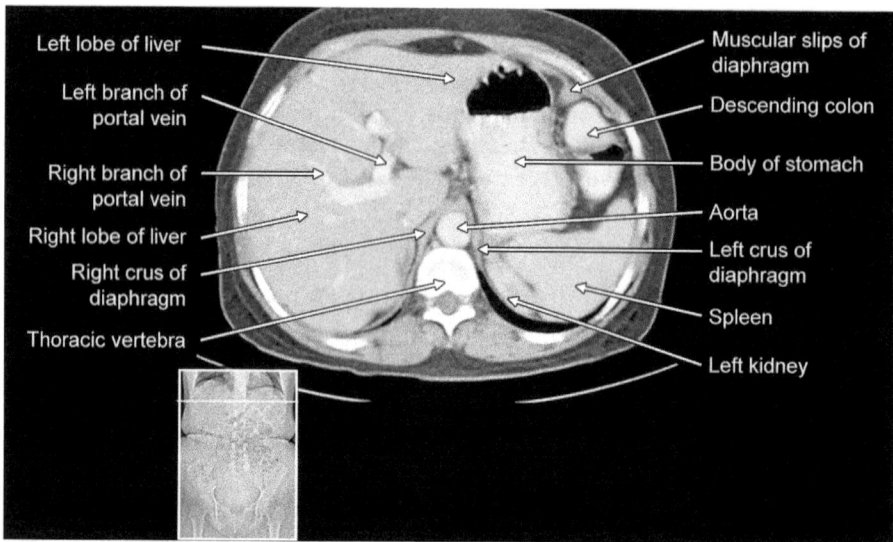

Fig. 8: Axial CT section of abdomen at the level of portal vein.

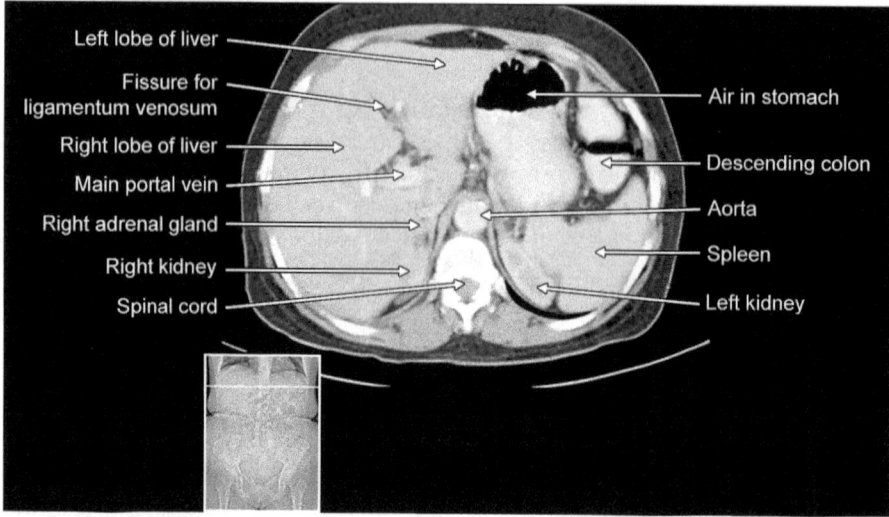

Fig. 9: Axial CT section of abdomen at the level of upper pole of both kidneys.

GASTROINTESTINAL SYSTEM

The gastrointestinal system originates from a pouch-like extension of yolk sac starting from 6 weeks of gestational age. The foregut is supplied by celiac artery, midgut by superior mesenteric artery and the hindgut by inferior mesenteric artery.

Upper gastrointestinal system starts from mouth and continues into oropharynx which continues into esophagus. Esophagus is a 25 cm long tubular structure which opens into the stomach via gastroesophageal junction. Parts of stomach are the fundus, body, greater and lesser curvatures, antrum and pylorus. Walls are 3-5 mm thick except in pylorus where it can be upto 7 mm thick **(Figs. 12 to 23)**.

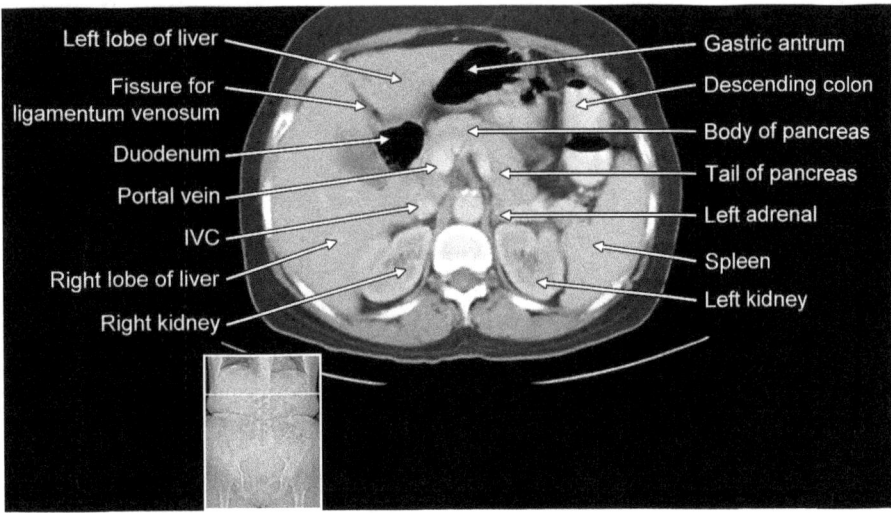

Fig. 10: Axial CT section of abdomen at the level of middle of both kidneys and body of pancreas.

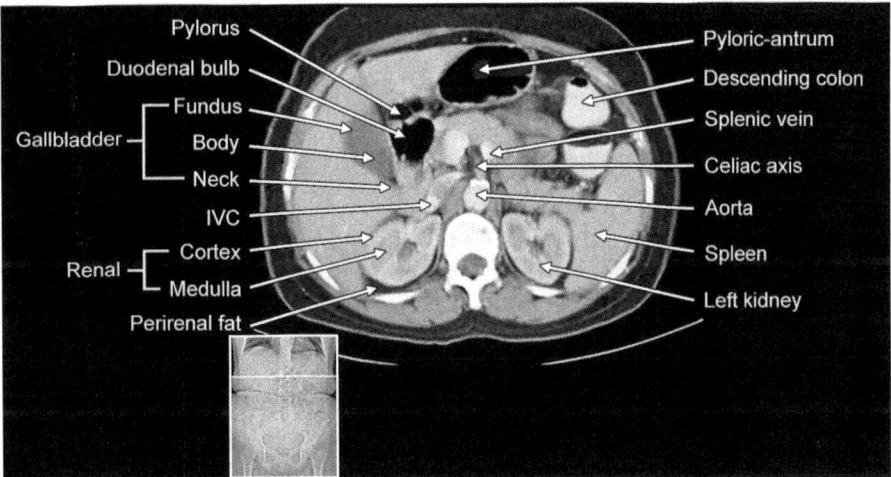

Fig. 11: Axial CT section of abdomen at the level of middle of gallbladder and pancreas.

Small intestine can be upto 6 m long and extends from pyloric orifice of stomach up to ileocecal valve. Duodenum is 1 feet long, jejunum is around 10 feet and ileum is upto 8 feet. Fifteen centimeters long mesentery is located between ileocecal junction and ligament of Treitz. Circular folds of small bowel are called valvulae conniventes.

Rule of three for normal small bowel states that its walls are 3 mm thick, valvulae conniventes are 3 mm thick, there are less than 3 air fluid levels and the diameter is upto 3 cm.

Large intestine is 1.5 m long and extends from distal to terminal ileum to anus. Its parts are cecum, ascending colon, hepatic flexure of colon, transverse colon, splenic flexure, descending colon, sigmoid colon, rectum and anal canal.

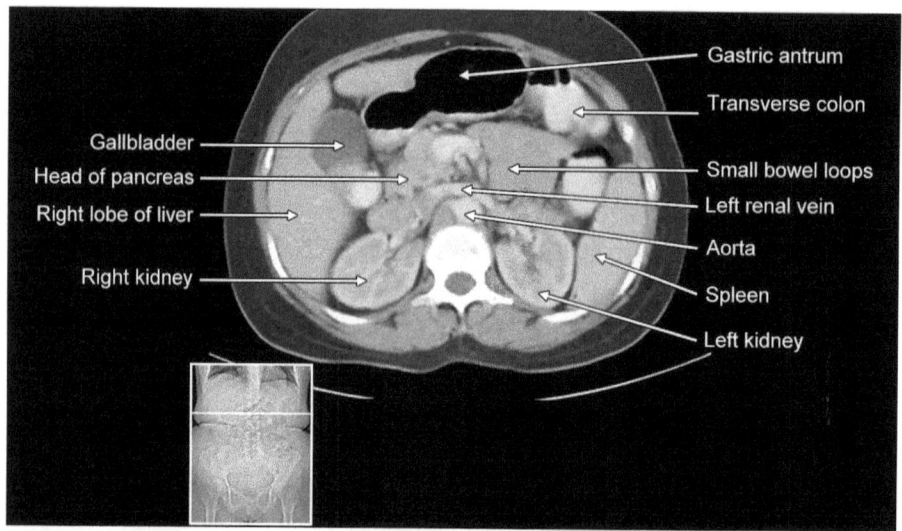

Fig. 12: Axial CT section of abdomen at the level of renal veins and head of pancreas.

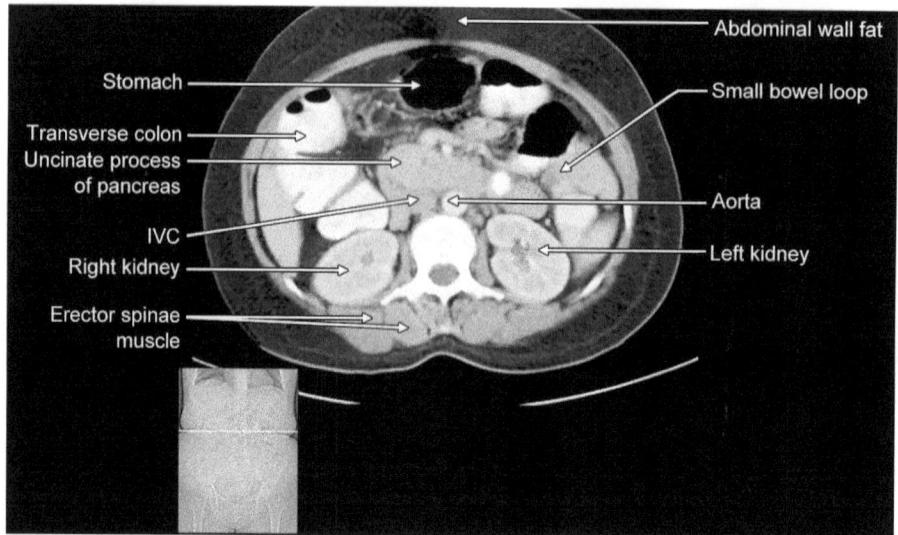

Fig. 13: Axial CT section of abdomen showing kidneys and uncinate process of pancreas.

Peritoneal spaces above transverse colon are:
- Spaces on the right
  - Right subphrenic space
  - Anterior and posterior right subhepatic space
  - Bare area of liver
  - Lesser sac
- Spaces on the left
  - Left subphrenic space
  - Left subhepatic space
  - Perisplenic space

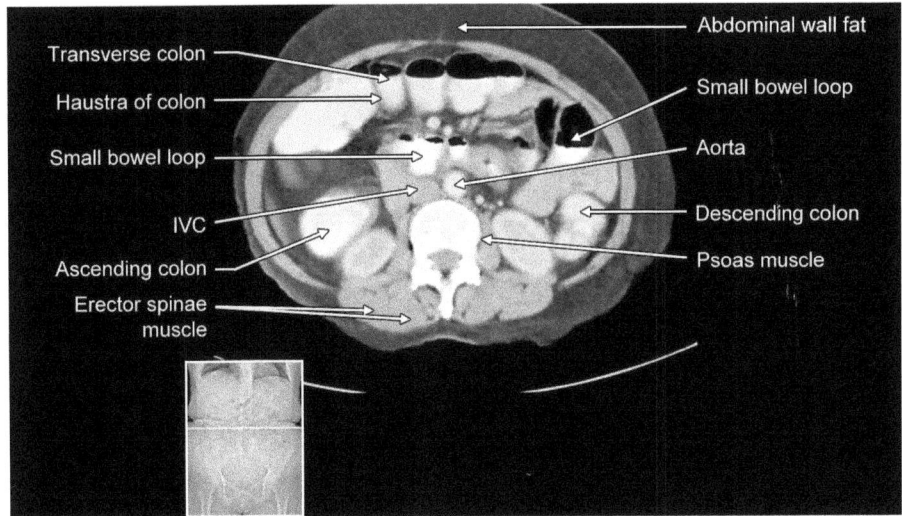

Fig. 14: Axial CT section of abdomen showing most of the colon.

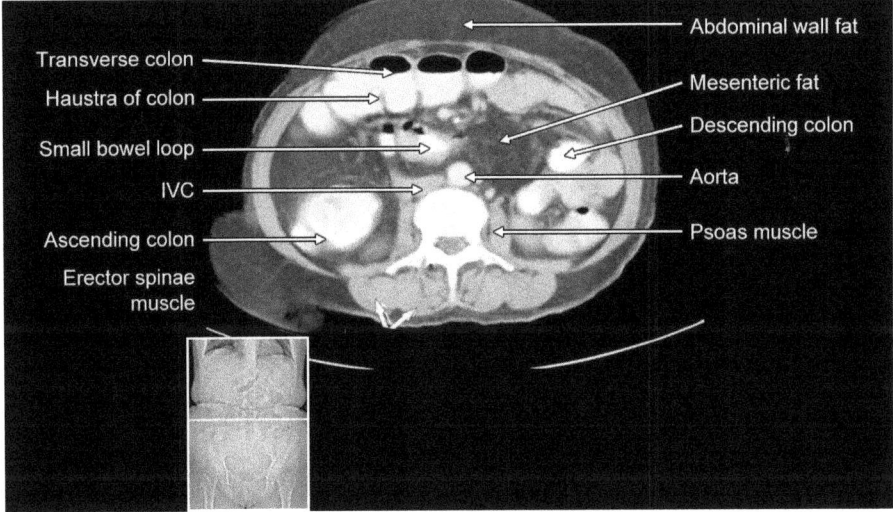

Fig. 15: Axial CT section of abdomen showing transverse colon with haustra.

Peritoneal spaces below transverse colon are:
- Superior and inferior ileocecal recesses
- Retrocecal space
- Right and left paracolic gutters
- Intersigmoid recess

Two folds of peritoneum supporting a structure within the peritoneal cavity together form a structure known as ligament.

When two folds of peritoneum connect a portion of bowel to the retroperitoneum it is known as mesentery. Ventral mesentery gives rise to falciform ligament, gastrohepatic ligament and hepatoduodenal ligament. Dorsal mesentery gives rise to gastrophrenic ligament,

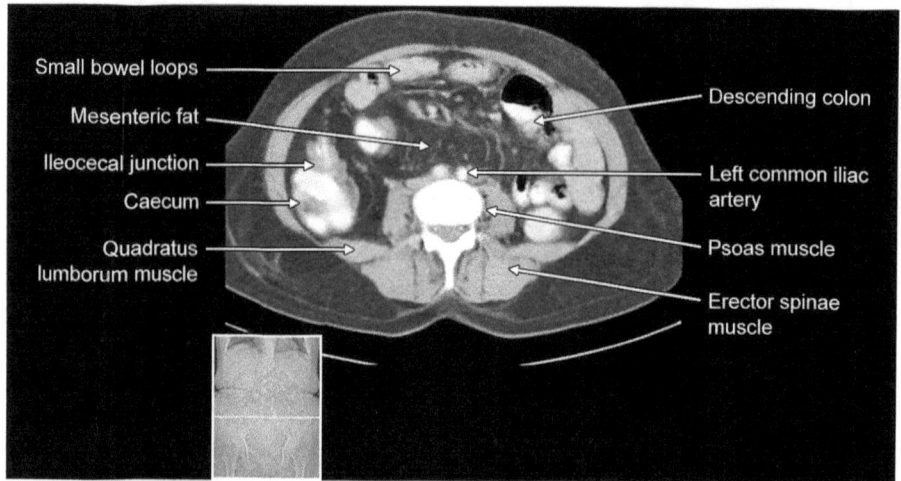

Fig. 16: Axial CT section of abdomen showing aortic bifurcation into iliac arteries.

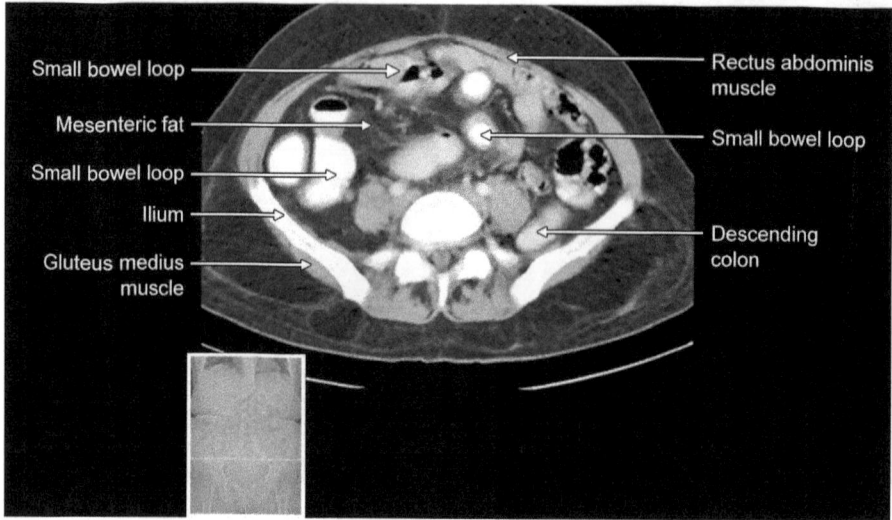

Fig. 17: Axial CT section of pelvis showing small bowel loops.

gastropancreatic ligament, phrenicocolic ligament, gastrosplenic ligament, splenorenal ligament and gastrocolic ligament. Dorsal mesentery also forms the small bowel mesentery and transverse as well as sigmoid mesocolons. Omentum is a structure connecting stomach to an additional structure. Lesser omentum is formed by combination of hepatoduodenal and gastrohepatic ligament. Greater omentum is an inferior continuation of gastrocolic ligament and is composed of four layers of peritoneum resulting from double reflection of dorsal mesogastrium.

Anterior right subhepatic space located posterior to porta hepatis communicates with lesser sac through epiploic foramen also known as foramen of Winslow.

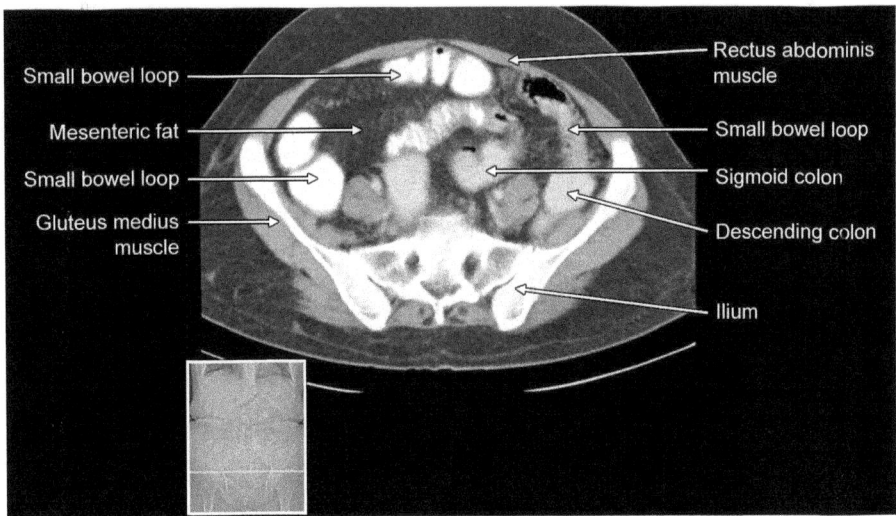

Fig. 18: Axial CT section of pelvis showing sigmoid colon.

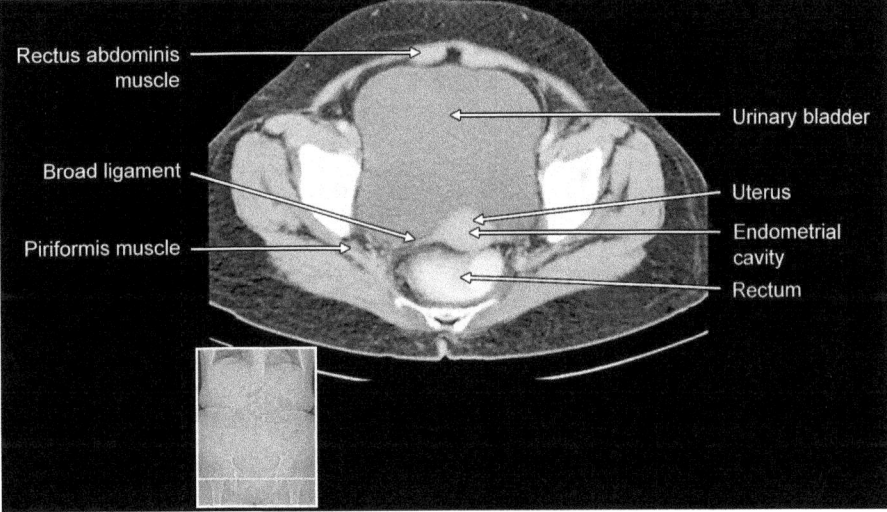

Fig. 19: Axial CT section of female pelvis showing uterus and broad ligament.

UROGENITAL SYSTEM

- Kidneys arise from metanephros (of mesodermal origin) at fourth week of intrauterine life. Bladder, urethra and prostate are formed from urogenital sinus.
- Adult kidneys have a span of 7-12 cm **(Figs. 10 to 13)**. Renal arteries arise from abdominal aorta at the level of L1-L2 vertebrae and then divide into following five segmental branches—apical, anterior superior, anterior inferior, posterior and basilar.

Section 1: Cross-Sectional Anatomy on CT Scan

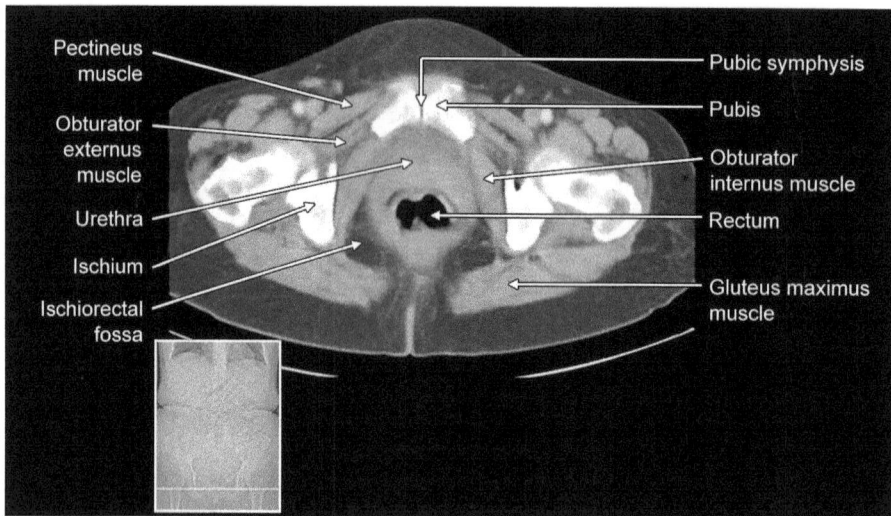

Fig. 20: Axial CT section of female pelvis showing pelvic muscles.

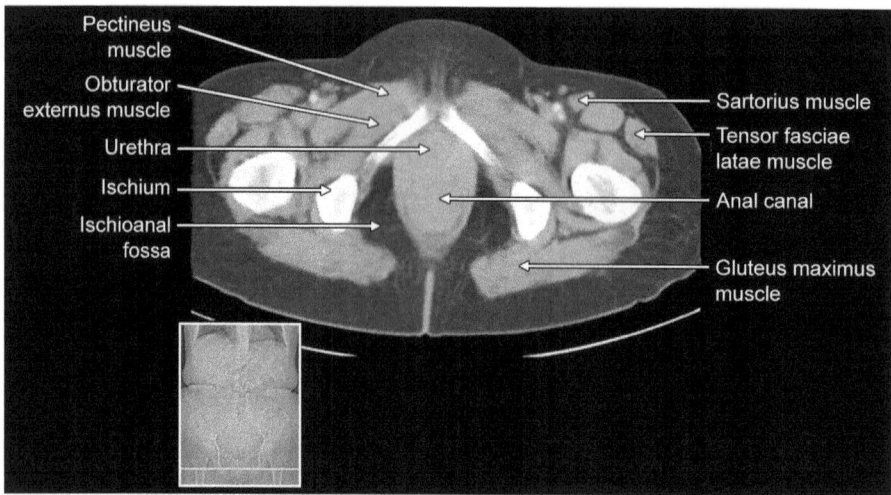

Fig. 21: Axial CT section of female pelvis showing urethra and anal canal.

- Renal arteries can be multiple, aberrant, accessory and even supplementary. Single or multiple renal veins can exist.
- Retroperitoneum is the space between parietal peritoneum extending from diaphragm to pelvic brim and fascia transversalis.
- Adrenal glands (suprarenal glands) are situated on the top of kidneys and are 3 cm long and 1 cm thick.
- Average size of testis is 2.5 × 3.0 × 3.5 cm. Epididymis has a head, body and a tail.
- Spermatic cord consists of testicular artery, cremasteric artery, pampiniform plexus of veins, vas deferens, nerves and lymphatics.

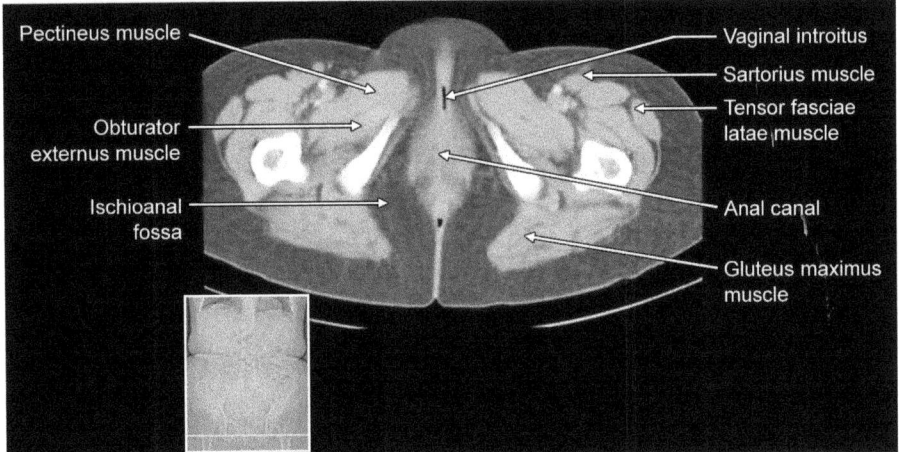

Fig. 22: Axial CT section of female pelvis showing vaginal introitus.

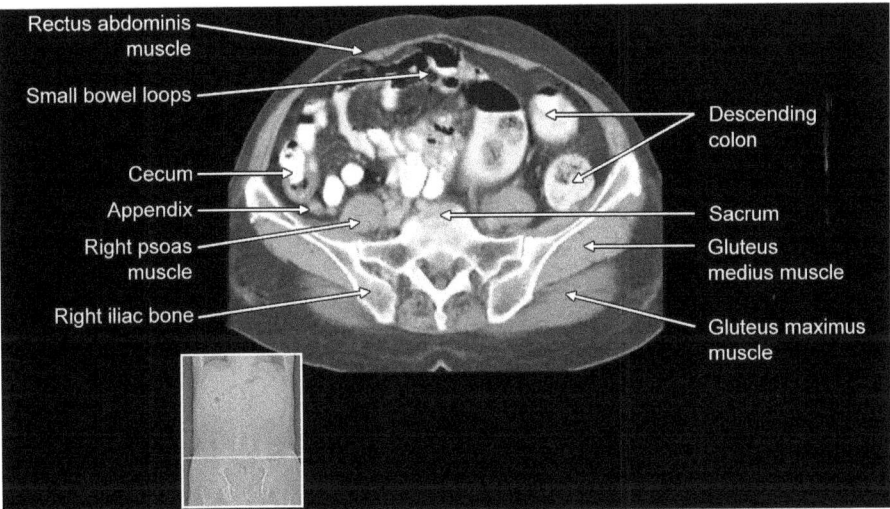

Fig. 23: Axial CT section at the level of appendix.

- Gonadal artery arises from ventral surface of aorta slightly below the origin of renal arteries. Occasionally it can arise from renal artery.
- Gonadal veins drain in the IVC or renal vein on right and in the renal vein on left.
- Prostate has a normal size of 2.5 × 2.8 × 3.0 cm **(Fig. 24)**. It is composed of an outer part having a central and peripheral zone and an inner part made of periurethral and transitional zone.
- Male urethra is 15–20 cm long and has a posterior part composed of prostatic urethra and membranous urethra. The anterior part of urethra is composed of bulbar and penile urethra **(Fig. 25)**.

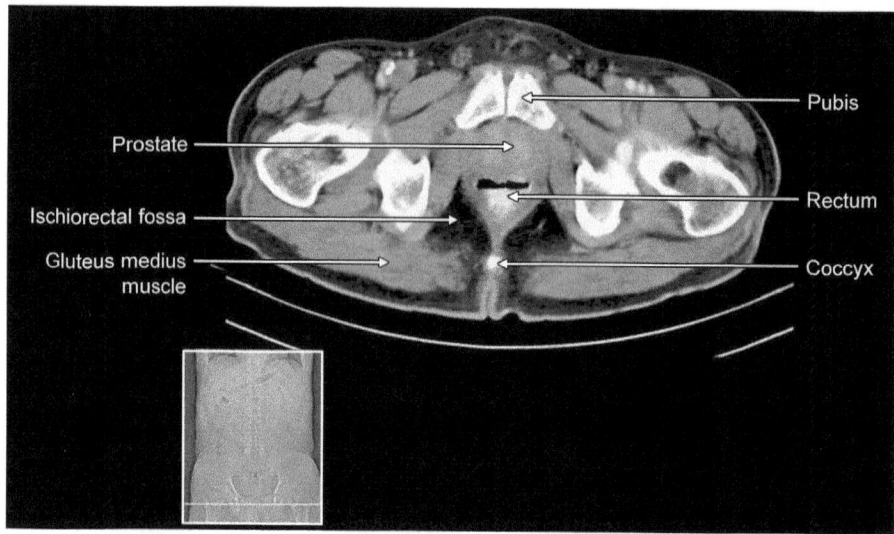

Fig. 24: Axial CT section of male pelvis showing prostate.

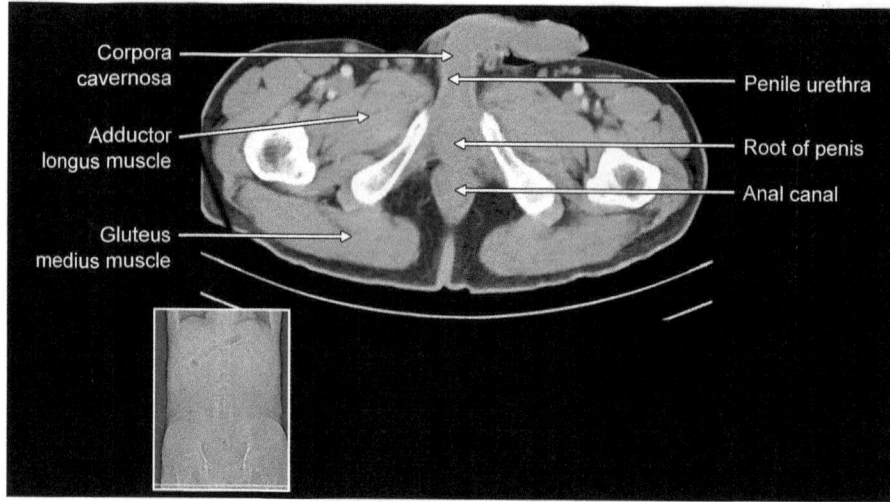

Fig. 25: Axial CT section of male pelvis showing penile anatomy.

- Female urethra is 2.5–5 cm Long
- Adult uterus is 6–9 cm long, 2.5–4 cm anteroposterior and 3–4.5 cm transverse in dimension **(Fig. 19)**. Endometrium is the innermost zone of uterus. Serosa is the outermost zone. Myometrium is the middle layer. CT scan usually does not show them separately.
- Fallopian tubes arise from upper and the outer aspect of uterus, and extend between the folds of broad ligament towards the pelvic side walls to open just above and anterior to ovaries located in ovarian fossa on each side.
- Pelvic spaces formed due to relationship between urinary bladder, uterus and rectum are:
  - Rectouterine pouch of Douglas

- Uterovesical pouch
- Rectovesical recess

Important pelvic ligaments in relation to uterus are:
- **Broad ligament:** Between uterus and pelvic sidewalls **(Fig. 19)**
- **Round ligament:** Between uterus and labia majora
- **Cardinal ligament/Mackenrodt ligament:** Between cervix and fascia of obturator internus
- **Uterosacral ligament:** Between uterus and sacrum
    Adult ovaries measure 1.0 cm × 2.0 cm × 3.0 cm.

CHAPTER 10

Joints of Upper Extremity

Upper extremity has three parts:
a. **Upper arm which has a bone:** Humerus.
b. **Forearm which has two bones:** Radius and ulna
c. **Wrist and hand:** Wrist has 8 carpals and hand has 5 metacarpals and 14 phalanges.

The upper limb is attached to the trunk by shoulder girdle which is made of scapula posteriorly and clavicle anteriorly.

SHOULDER JOINT

It is a ball and socket type synovial joint formed by glenoid of scapula and head of humerus (**Figs. 1 to 8**). Humeral head is large and broad than glenoid cavity due to which this joint is intrinsically weak. Hence to provide stability to this joint, it is surrounded by rotator cuff made of muscles and tendons and coracoacromial arch made of coracoid process, acromion, coracoacromial ligament and acromioclavicular joint. Strong superior, middle and inferior glenohumeral capsular ligaments also impart glenohumeral stability.

Rotator cuff is formed by subscapularis, supraspinatus, infraspinatus and teres minor arranged antero-posteriorly.

Complex intra-articular fractures and fractures of scapula can particularly be seen in great details by CT scan.

ELBOW JOINT

Distal articulating surface of humerus and proximal articulating surfaces of radius and ulna participate in forming this synovial joint (**Figs. 9 to 17**). Radial head is aligned in place against radial notch of ulna by annular ligament. Radial collateral ligament and ulnar collateral ligament also help keeping elbow in reduction. Triceps is the main extensor and biceps is the secondary supinator of elbow.

CT is particularly useful in detecting subtle fractures, loose bodies and the extent of heterotopic bone formation in and around elbow joint.

WRIST JOINT

Radiocarpal and distal radioulnar joints together form the wrist joint (**Figs. 18 to 23**). Subtle fractures and dislocations of carpals like scaphoid and lunate and distal radioulnar dislocations are best seen on CT scan even though plain radiographs may appear normal. Persistent pain on radial aspect of palm particularly in golfers is usually due to fracture of hook of hamate and is best shown by CT scan.

Chapter 10: Joints of Upper Extremity

CT SHOULDER

NORMAL ANATOMY

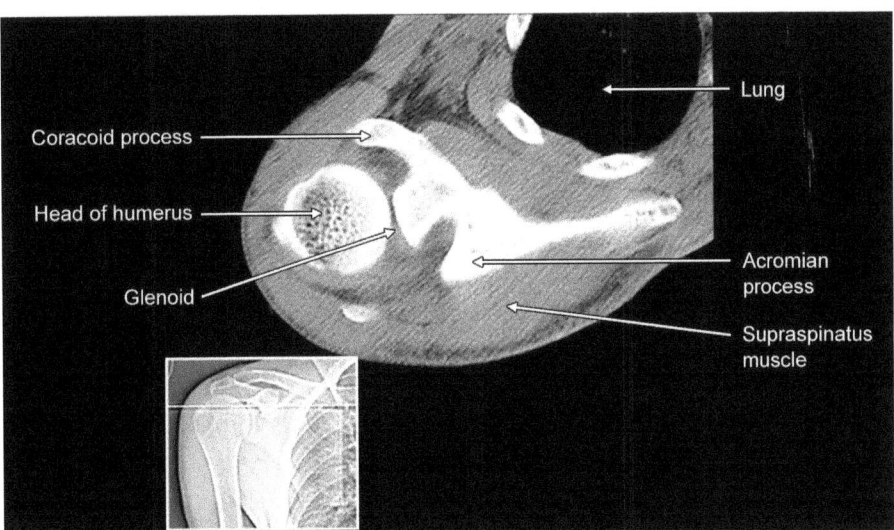

Fig. 1: Axial CT section of shoulder, level superior part of head of humerus.

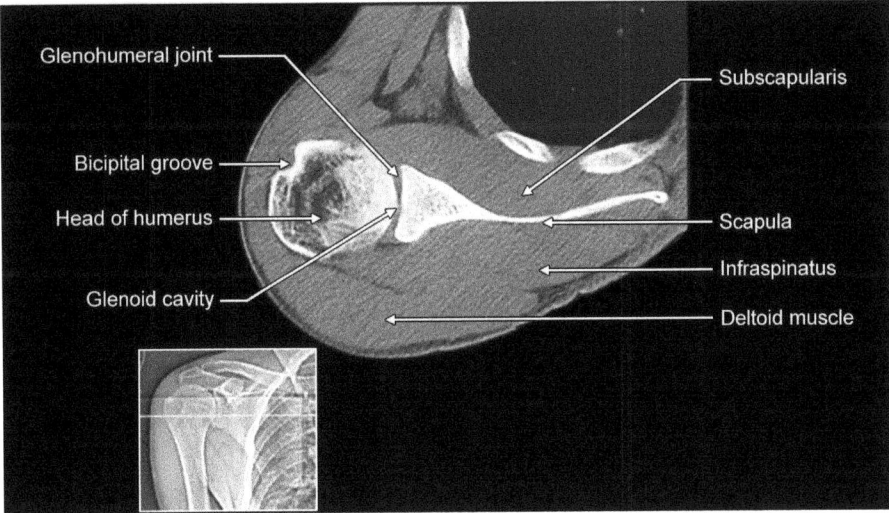

Fig. 2: Axial CT section of shoulder, level middle part of head of humerus.

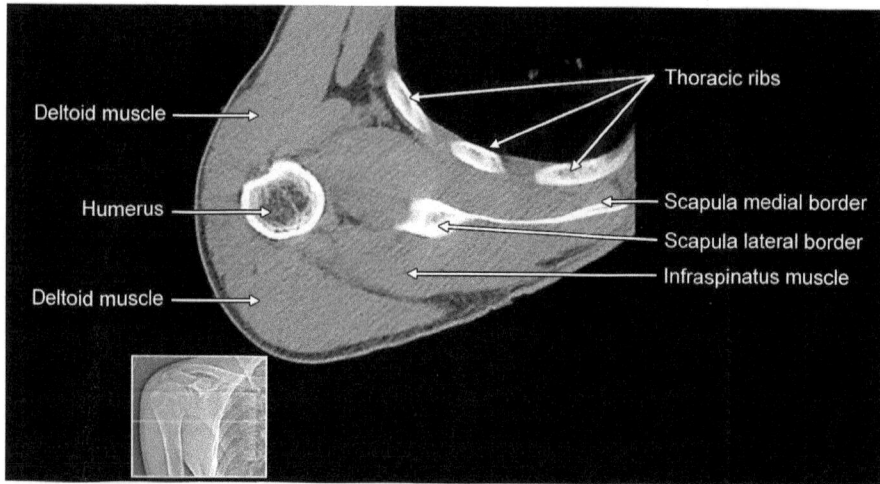

Fig. 3: Axial CT section of shoulder, level proximal part of shaft of humerus.

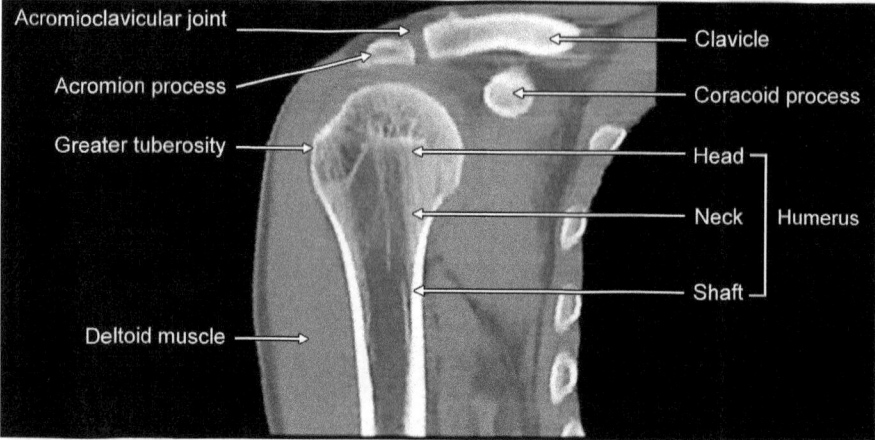

Fig. 4: Coronal recon of shoulder through head of humerus.

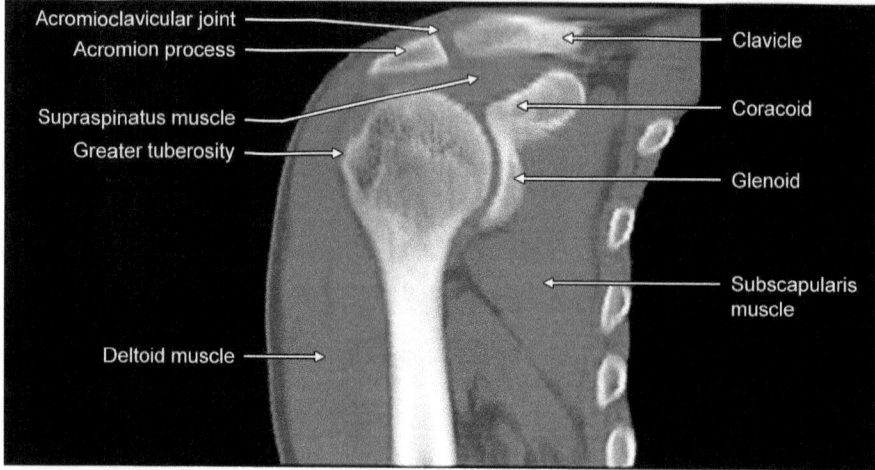

Fig. 5: Coronal recon of shoulder showing glenohumeral joint.

Chapter 10: Joints of Upper Extremity

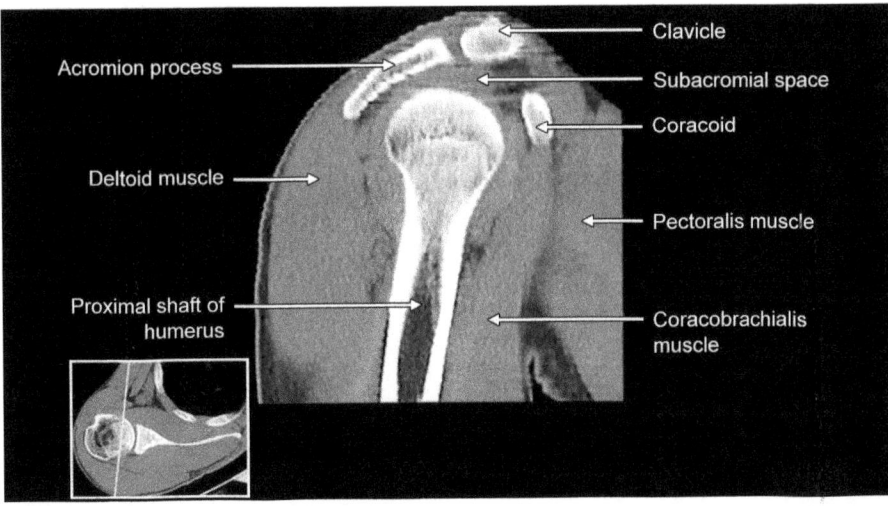

Fig. 6: Sagittal recon of shoulder joint.

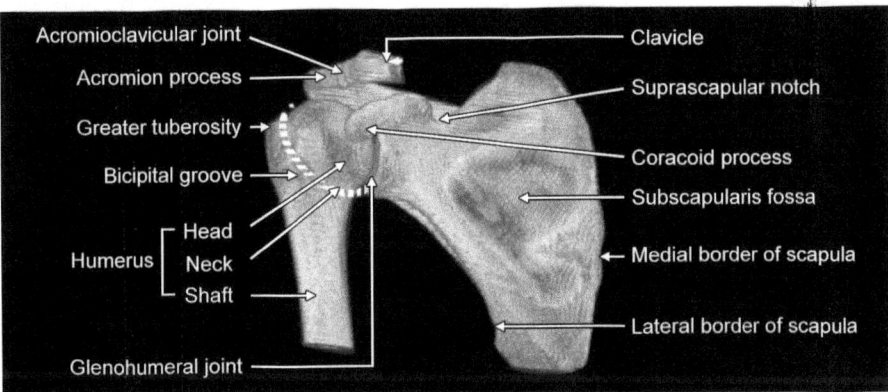

Fig. 7: Volume rendered 3D recon of shoulder (anteroposterior projection).

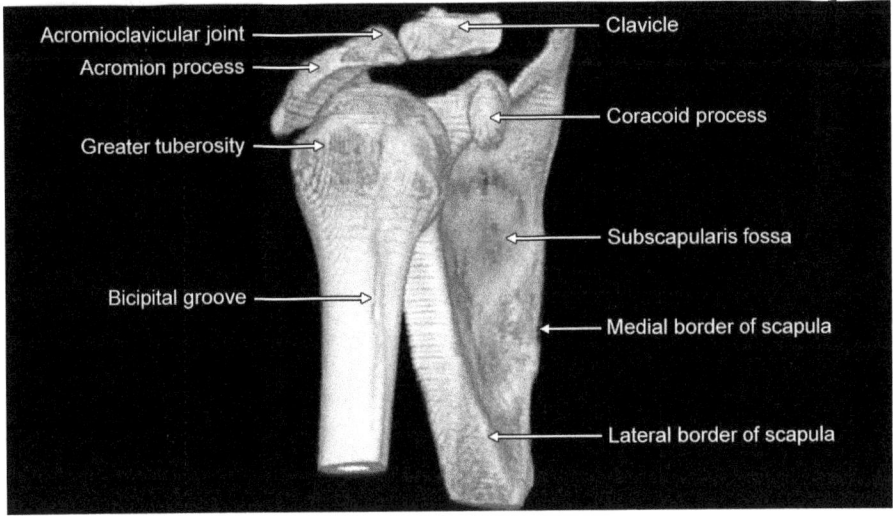

Fig. 8: Volume rendered 3D recon of shoulder (lateral oblique projection).

CT ELBOW JOINT

NORMAL ANATOMY

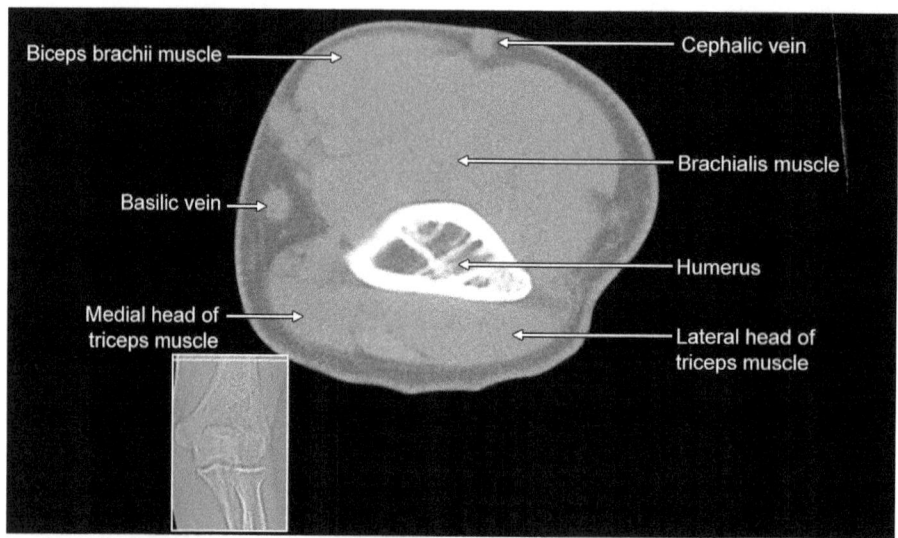

Fig. 9: Axial CT section of elbow, level distal shaft of humerus.

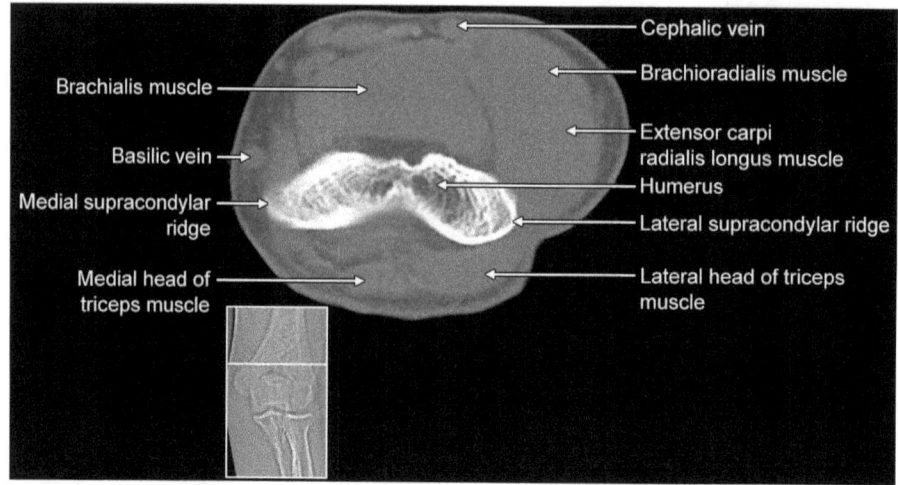

Fig. 10: Axial CT section of elbow, level supracondylar ridge of humerus.

Chapter 10: Joints of Upper Extremity

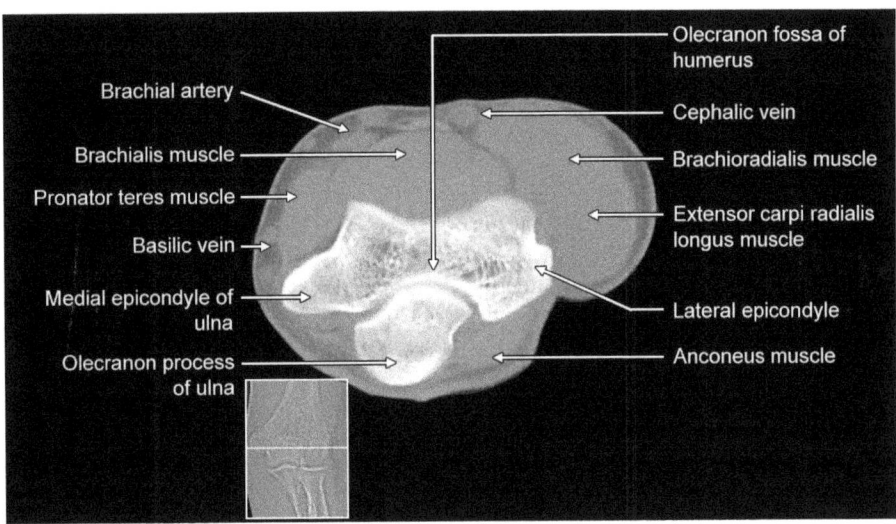

Fig. 11: Axial CT section of elbow, level epicondyles of humerus.

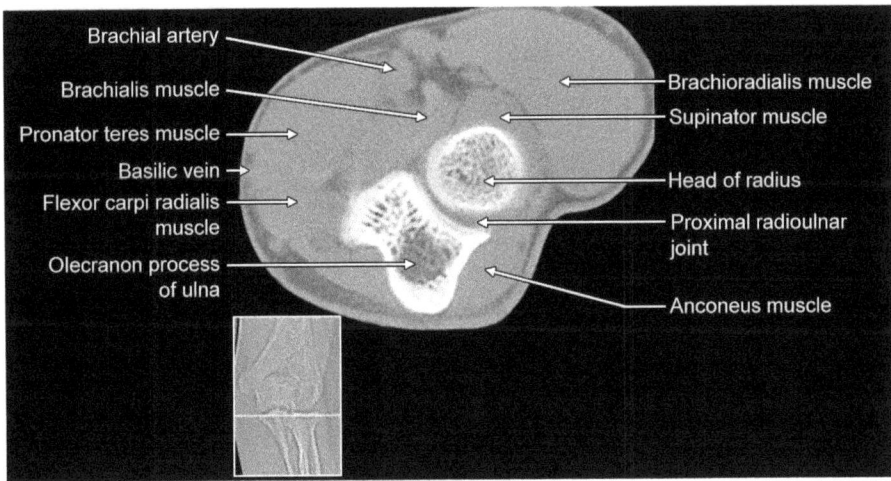

Fig. 12: Axial CT section of elbow, level head of radius.

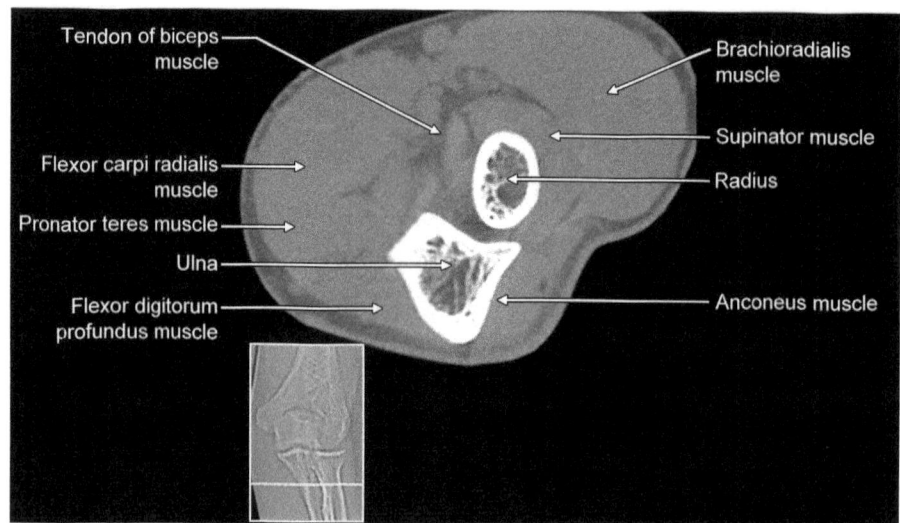

Fig. 13: Axial CT section of elbow, level proximal shaft of ulna and radius.

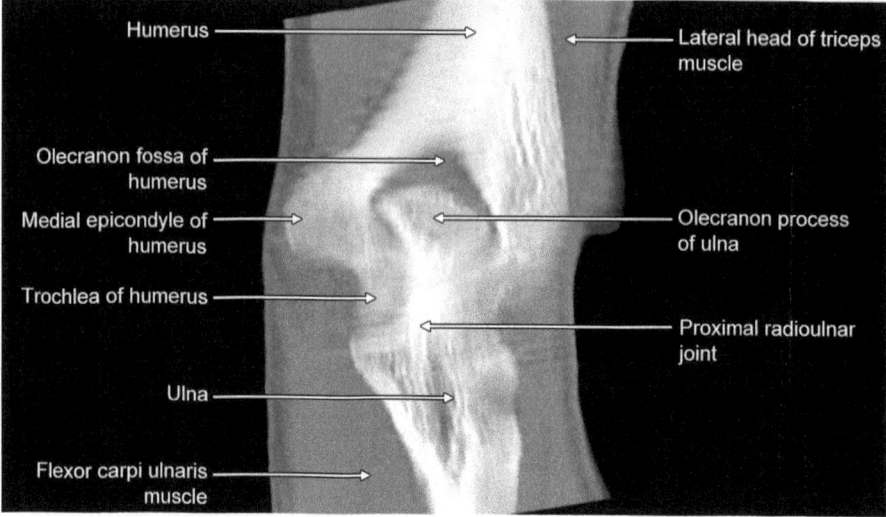

Fig. 14: Coronal CT recon of elbow joint and proximal radioulnar joint.

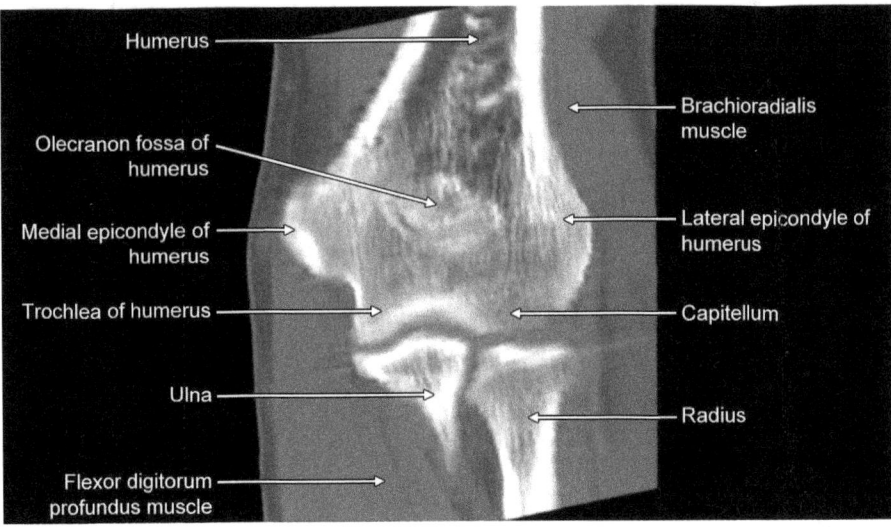

Fig. 15: Coronal CT recon of elbow showing humeroradial and humeroulnar articulation.

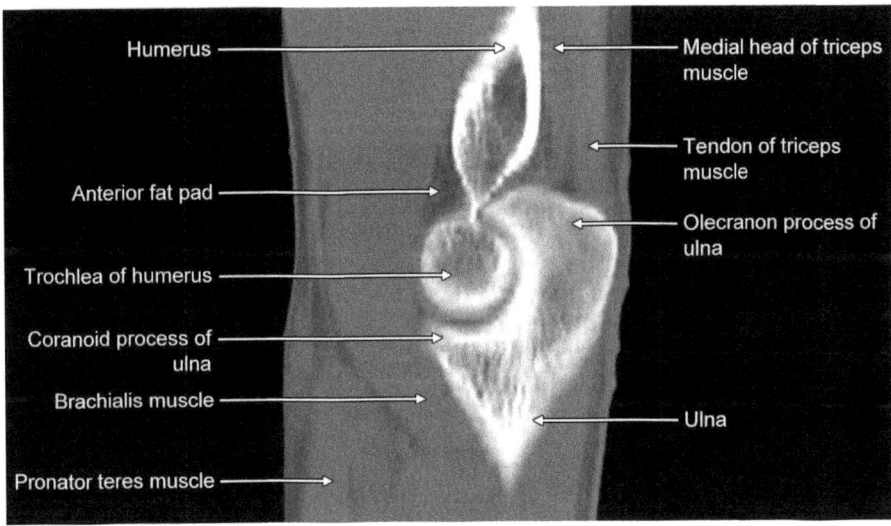

Fig. 16: Sagittal CT recon of elbow through humeroulnar joint.

Section 1: Cross-Sectional Anatomy on CT Scan

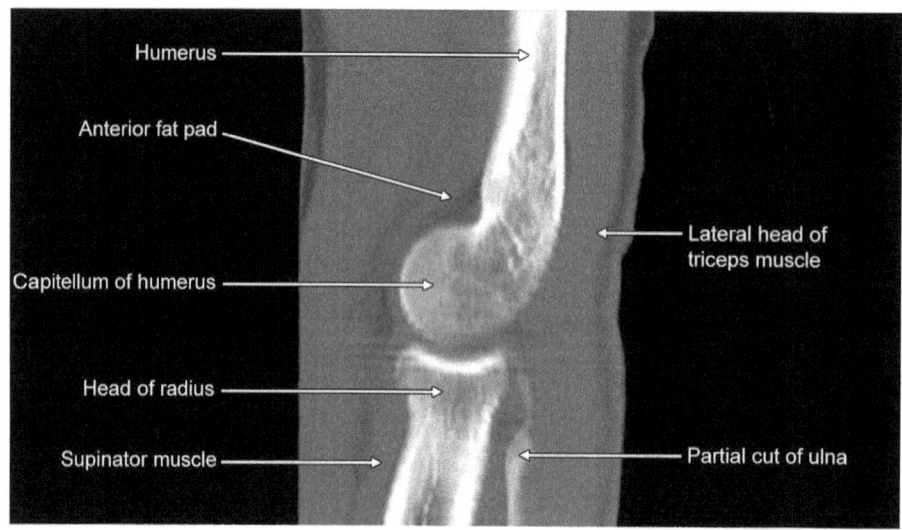

Fig. 17: Sagittal CT recon of elbow showing radio-capitellum joint.

CT WRIST

NORMAL ANATOMY

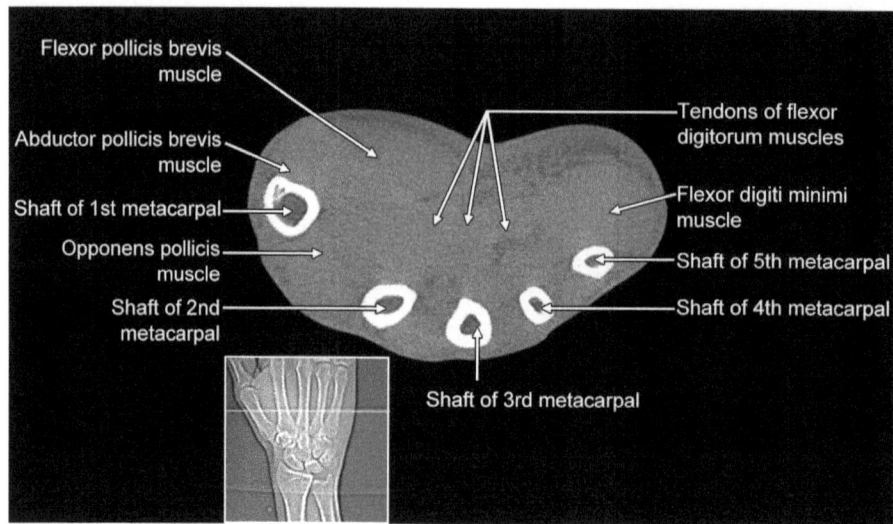

Fig. 18: Axial CT section of wrist at the level of proximal metacarpal.

Chapter 10: Joints of Upper Extremity

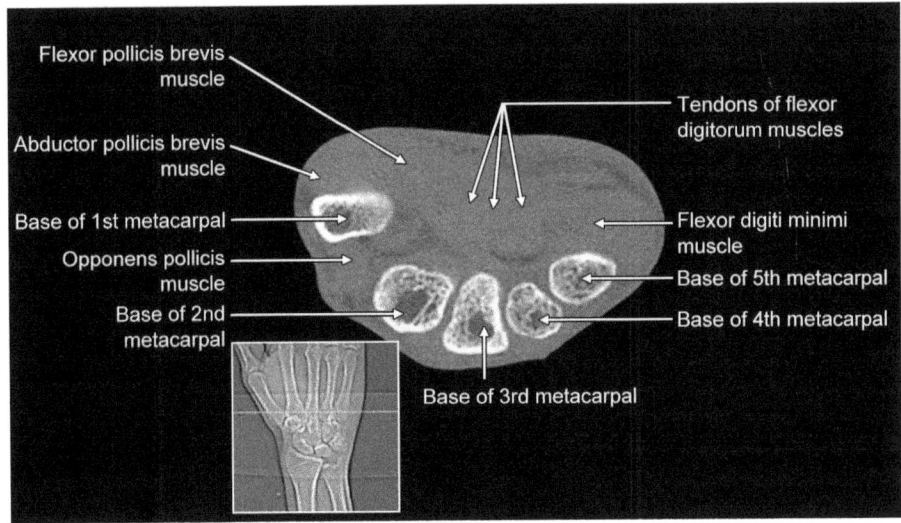

Fig. 19: Axial CT section of wrist at the level of bases of metacarpal.

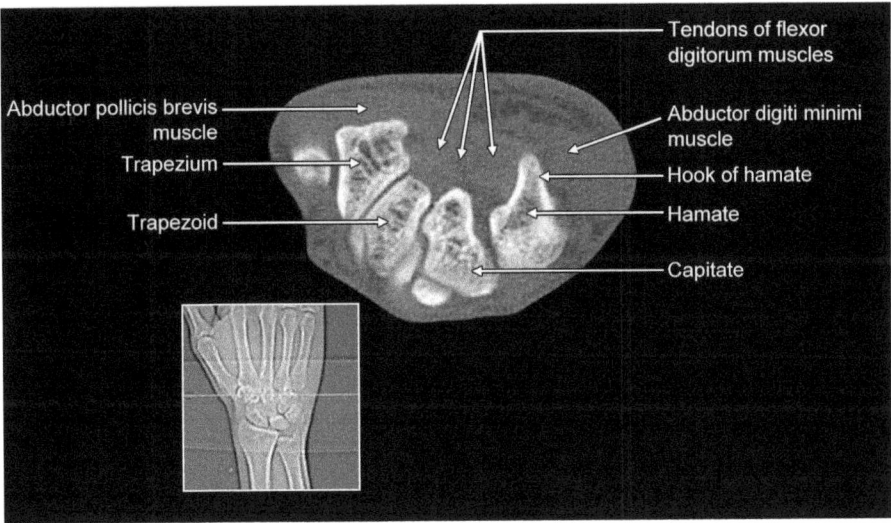

Fig. 20: Axial CT section of wrist at the level of distal row of carpel bones.

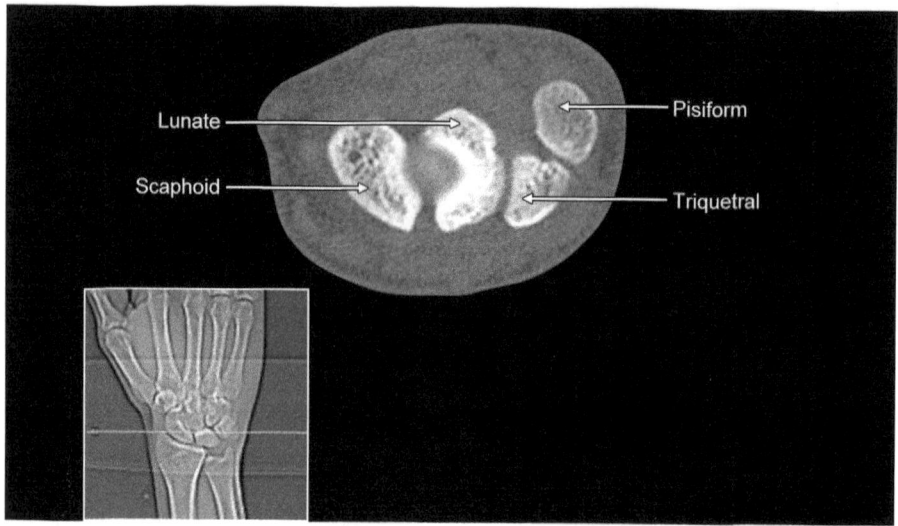

Fig. 21: Axial CT section of wrist at the level of proximal row of carpel bones.

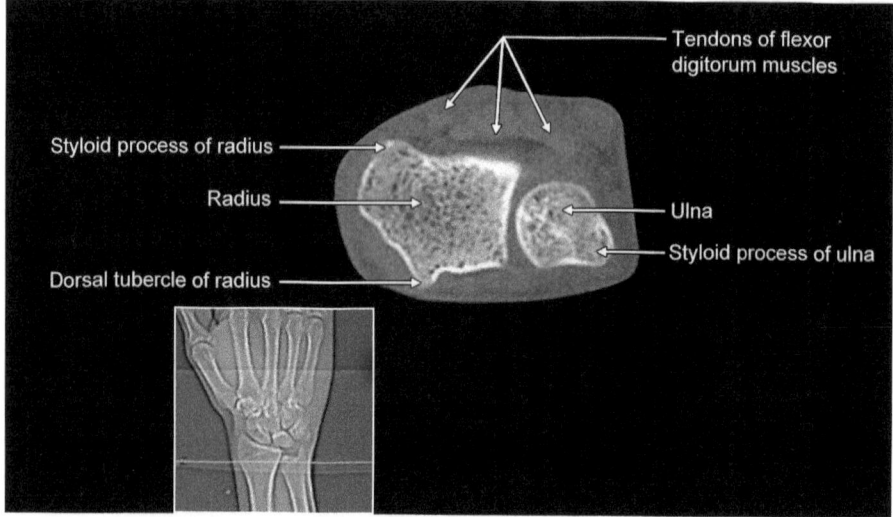

Fig. 22: Axial CT section of wrist at the level of styloid processes of radius and ulna.

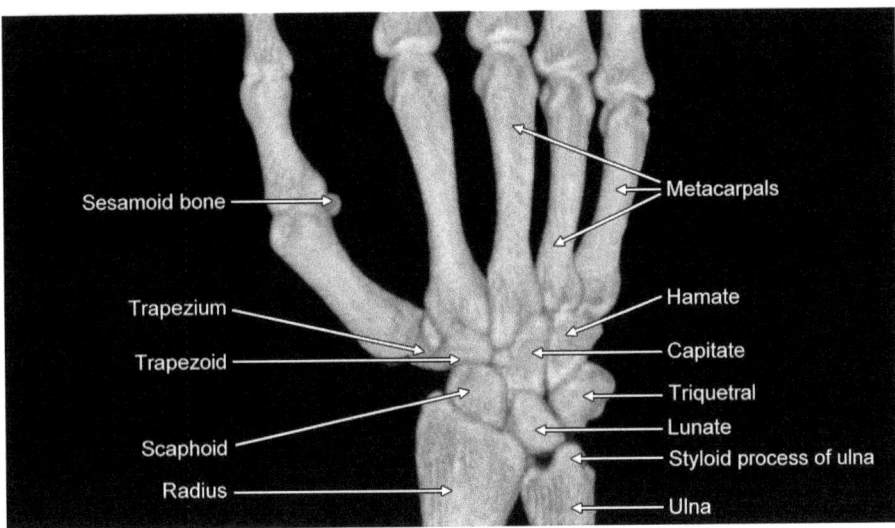

Fig. 23: Volume rendered 3D recon of wrist and hand.

CHAPTER 11

Joints of Lower Extremity

Lower extremity has three parts:
a. Thigh has a bone called femur which is the longest and strongest bone in the body.
b. Leg has two bones known as tibia and fibula.
c. Ankle has 7 tarsals. The foot contains 5 metatarsals and 14 phalanges.

The pelvis is a ring of bones situated between lower part of vertebral column and the lower limb. Posteriorly it is formed by sacrum and anterolaterally by two hip bones. Each hip bone has three portions called ilium, ischium and pubis.

HIP JOINT

It is a complex ball and socket type of synovial joint formed by femoral head, acetabulum, soft tissues, muscles and cartilages (**Figs. 1 to 6**). CT scan of hip joint followed by reformations in various planes provides exquisite details in multiple planes for an ideal three-dimensional perspective. Complex acetabular fractures and loose bodies or bone fragments are best seen on CT scan.

KNEE JOINT

Distal articulating surface of femur and proximal articulating surfaces of tibia and fibula participate in forming this synovial joint (**Figs. 7 to 16**). The tibiofemoral articulation is the main component of knee joint and is made stable by anterior and posterior cruciate ligaments and medial and lateral collateral ligaments. Joint surfaces are separated by medial and lateral menisci for shock absorption. Patellofemoral articulation imparts better leverage to quadriceps movement thereby further strengthening it.

Complex multiplanar fractures and loose bodies are best seen by CT scan.

FOOT AND ANKLE JOINTS

Ankle joint is formed between distal articulating surfaces of tibia-fibula–and-proximal articulating surface of talus (**Figs. 17 to 23**). Foot is divided into hindfoot (talus and calcaneum), midfoot (navicular bone, cuboid and three cuneiform bones) and forefoot (five metatarsals and three phalanges in each toe with only two phalanges in great toe).

Fracture patterns of calcaneum and talus can be well demonstrated by CT scan. Tarsal coalition, osteochondral lesions and various plantar arch deformities are also well seen.

Chapter 11: Joints of Lower Extremity

CT SECTIONS HIP JOINTS

NORMAL ANATOMY

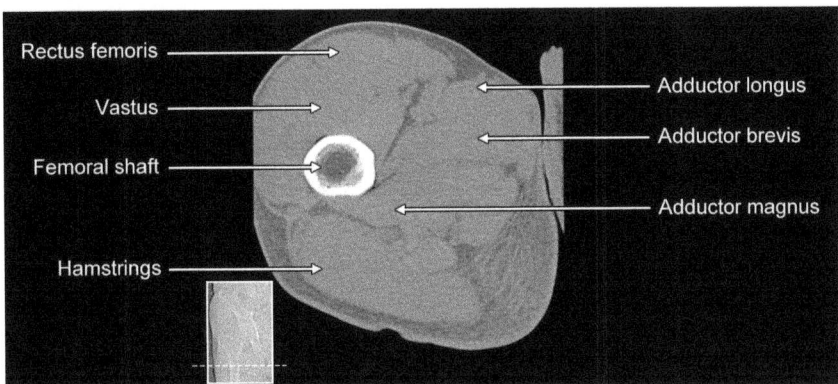

Fig. 1: Axial CT section at the level of proximal shaft of femur.

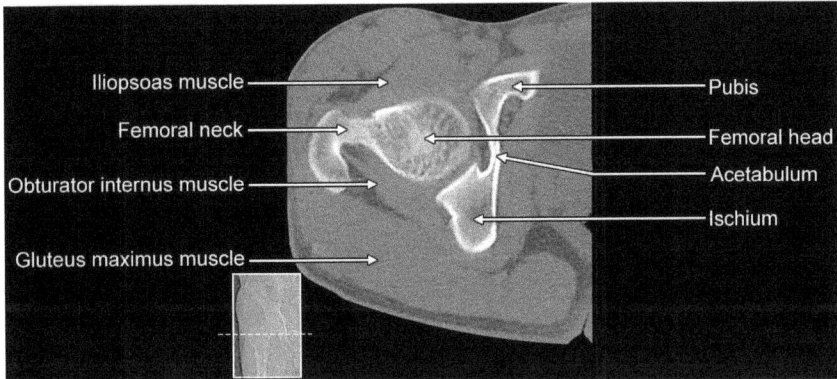

Fig. 2: Axial CT section at the level of hip joint.

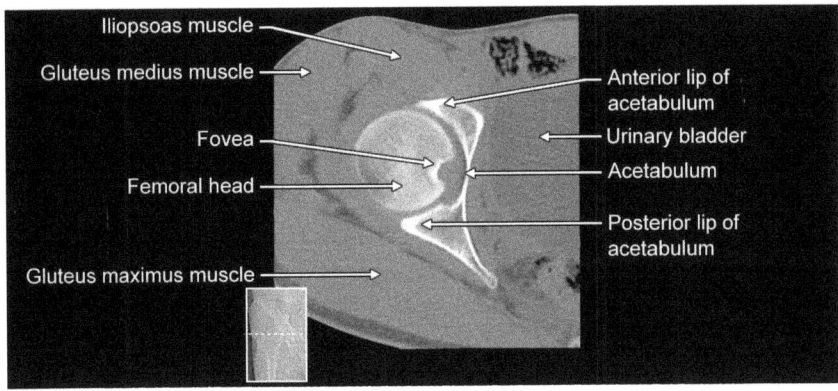

Fig. 3: Axial CT section of hip at the level of fovea of head of femur.

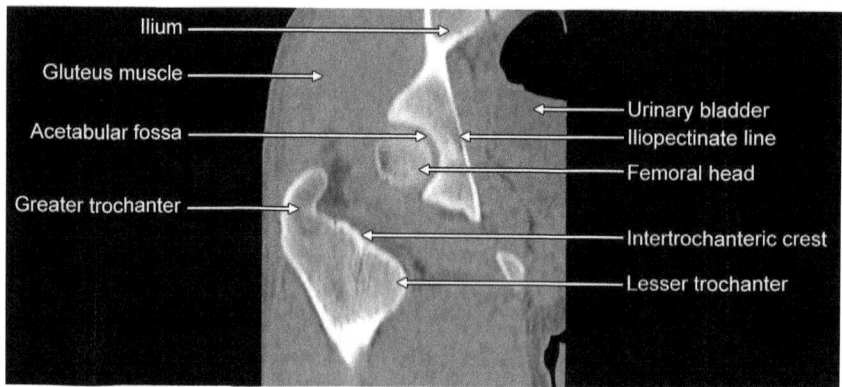

Fig. 4: Coronal CT recon of hip at the level of superior part of hip joint.

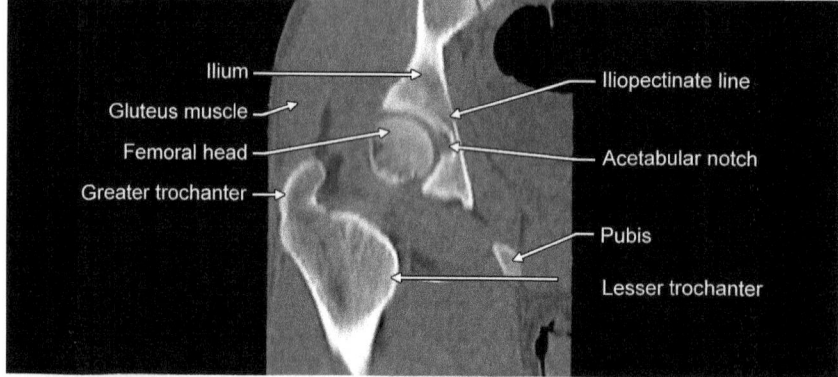

Fig. 5: Coronal CT reconstruction of hip at the level of acetabular notch.

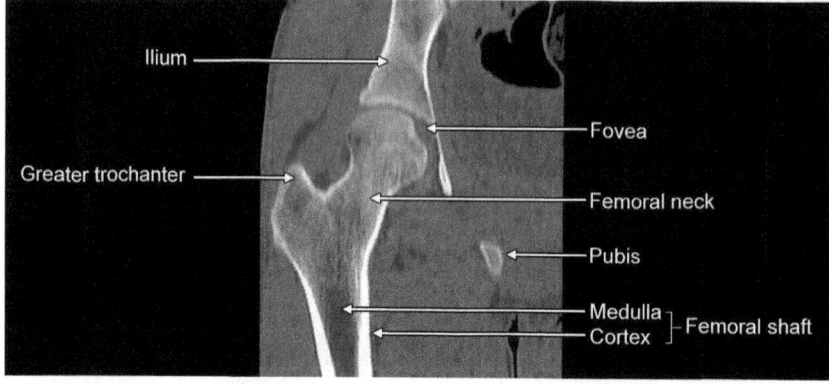

Fig. 6: Coronal CT reconstruction of hip.

Chapter 11: Joints of Lower Extremity

CT SECTION KNEE JOINT

NORMAL ANATOMY

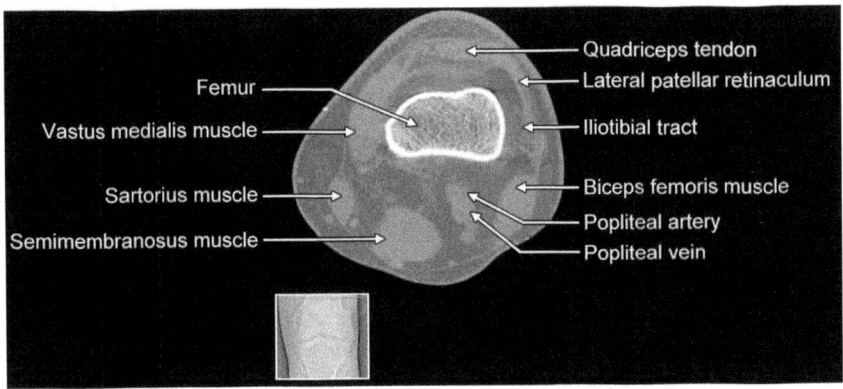

Fig. 7: Axial CT section of knee at the level of distal femur.

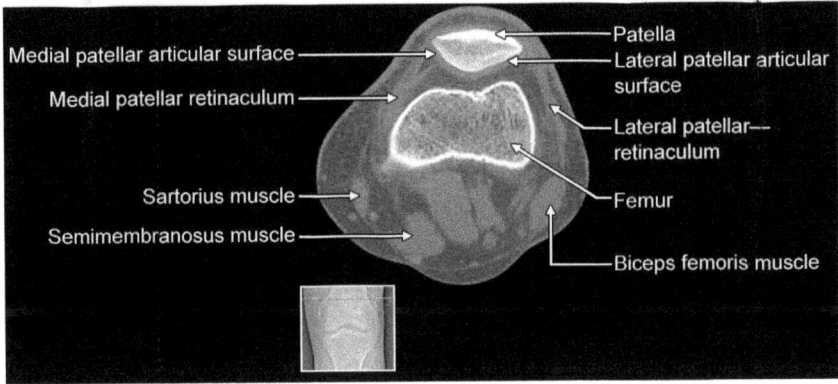

Fig. 8: Axial CT section of knee at the level of patella.

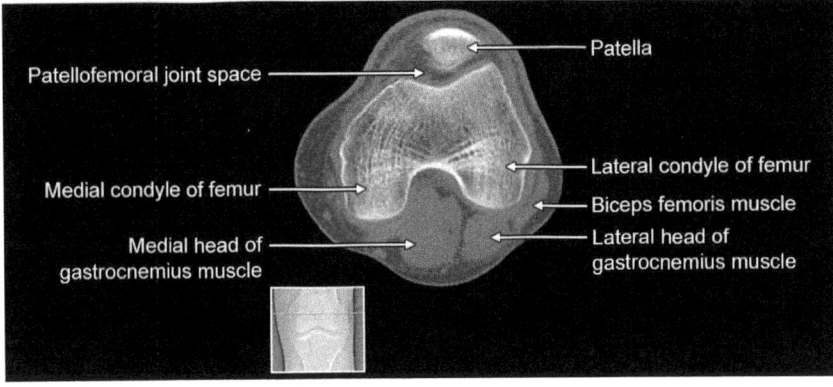

Fig. 9: Axial CT section of knee at the level of femoral condyles.

Section 1: Cross-Sectional Anatomy on CT Scan

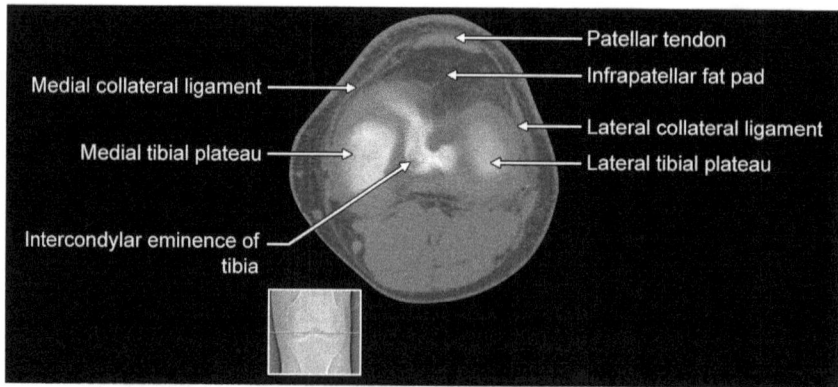

Fig. 10: Axial CT section of knee at the level of intercondylar eminence of tibia.

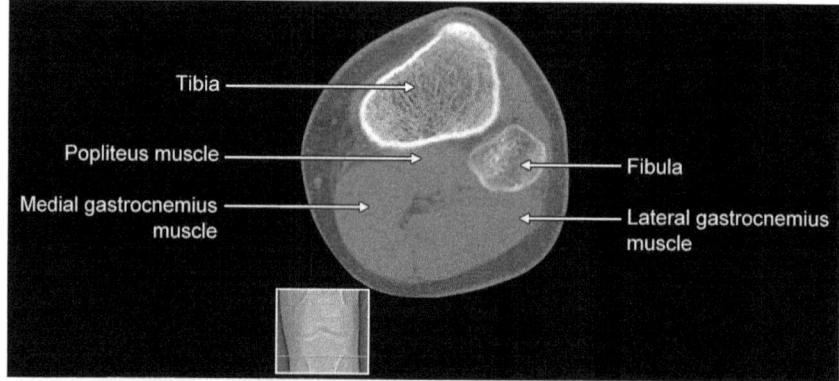

Fig. 11: Axial CT section of knee at the level of proximal part of tibia and fibula.

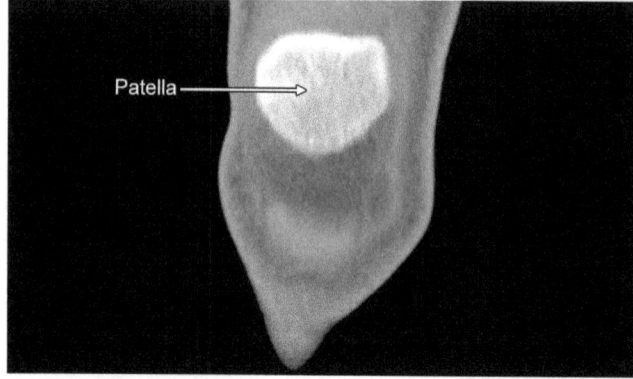

Fig. 12: Coronal CT recon of knee showing patella.

Chapter 11: Joints of Lower Extremity

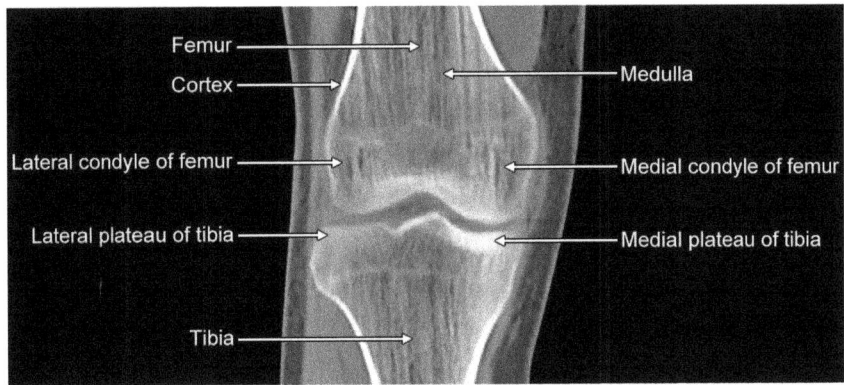

Fig. 13: Coronal CT recon of knee showing the knee joint being formed by tibia and fibula.

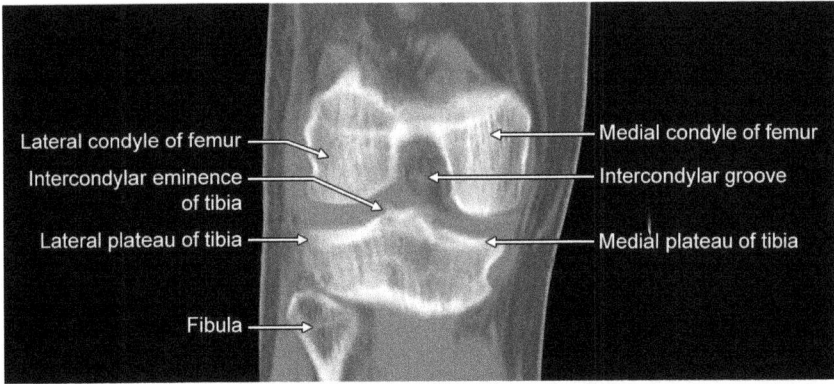

Fig. 14: Coronal CT recon of knee at the level of intercondylar eminence of fibula.

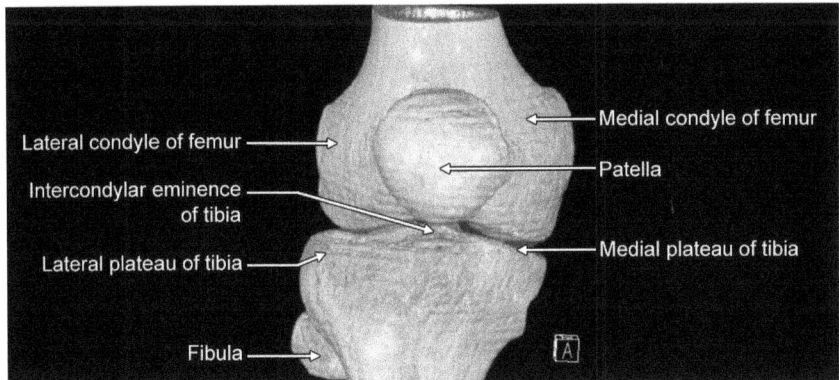

Fig 15: Volume rendered 3D CT recon of knee (anteroposterior projection).

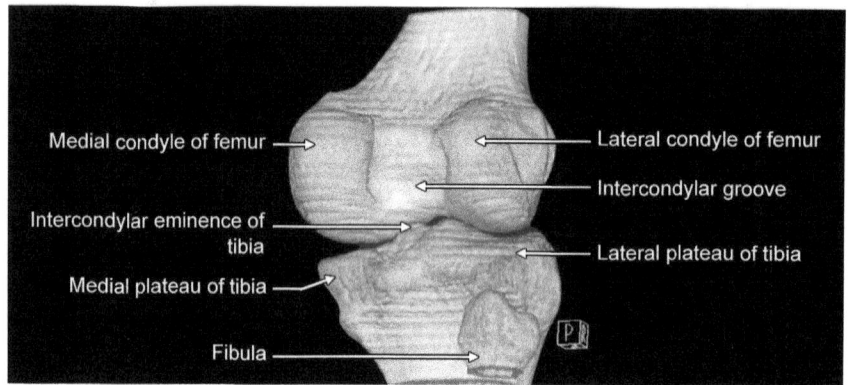

Fig. 16: Volume rendered 3D CT recon of knee (posteroanterior oblique projection).

CT SECTIONS FOOT AND ANKLE JOINT

NORMAL ANATOMY

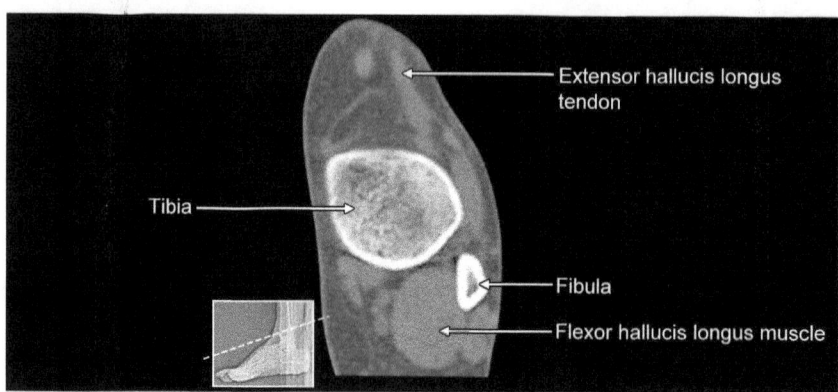

Fig. 17: Axial CT section of foot at the level of distal shaft of tibia and fibula.

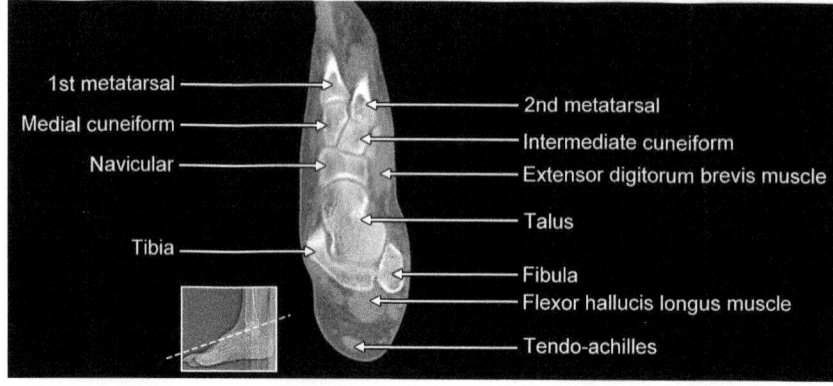

Fig. 18: Axial CT section of foot at the level of tarsal bones.

Chapter 11: Joints of Lower Extremity

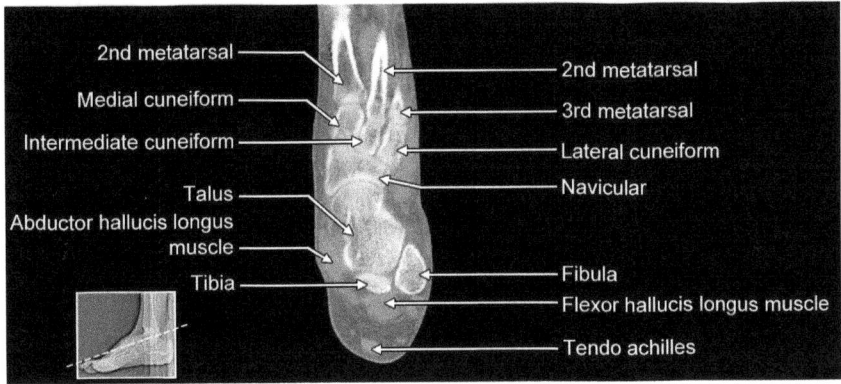

Fig. 19: Axial CT section of foot at the level of talus.

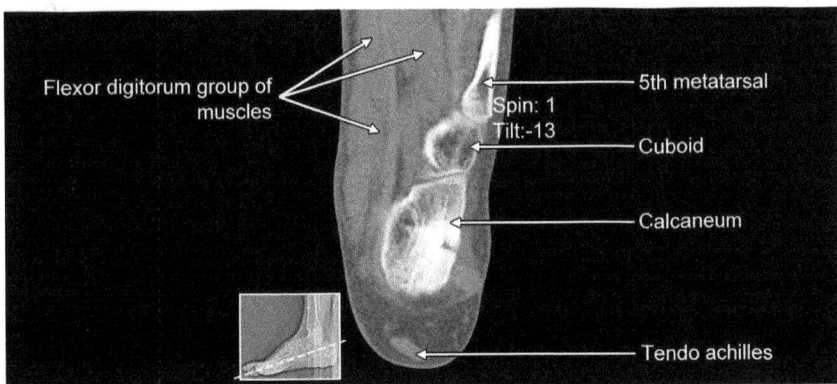

Fig. 20: Axial CT section of foot at the level of calcaneum.

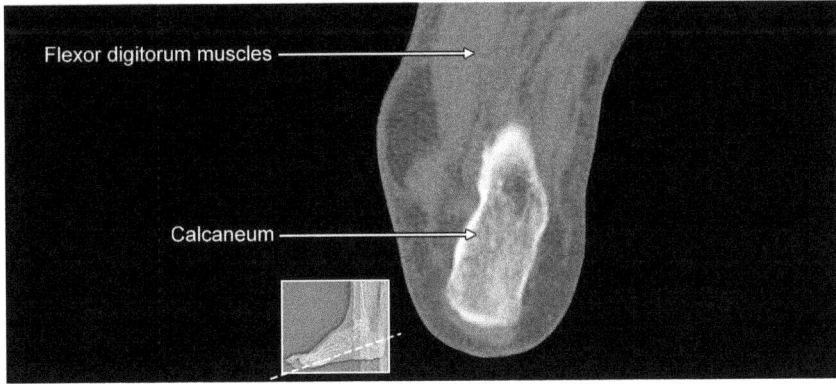

Fig. 21: Axial CT section of foot through the entire calcaneum.

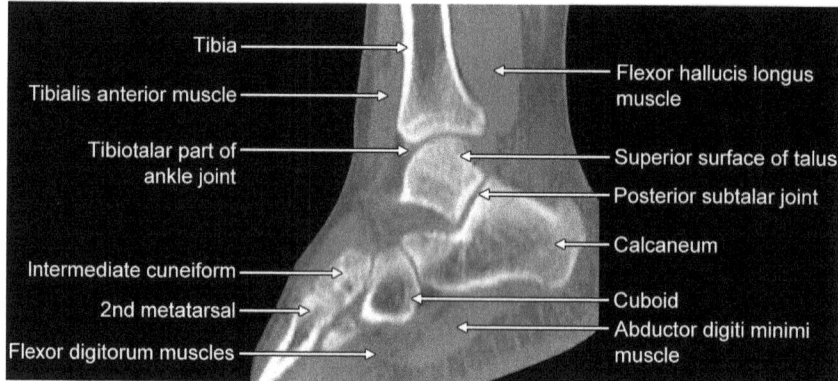

Fig. 22: Sagittal CT recon of foot showing calcaneum and cuboid bones.

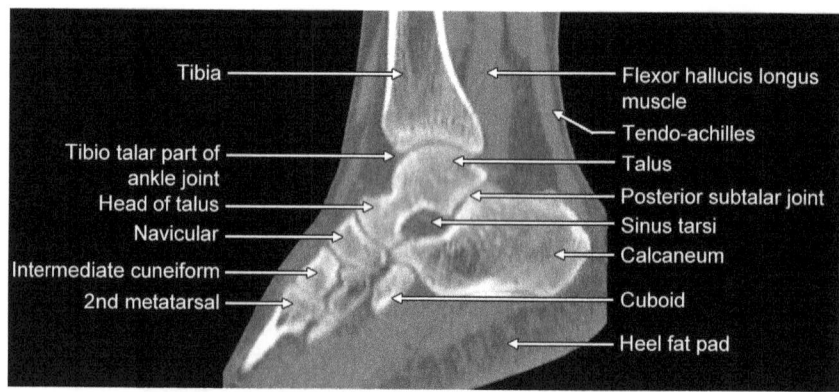

Fig. 23: Sagittal CT recon of foot showing most tarsal bones.

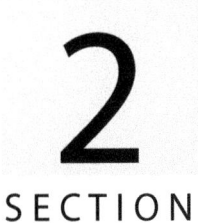

SECTION 2

EQUIPMENT, PHYSICS AND PROCEDURES

SECTION OUTLINE

- **Chapter 12:** Radiography and Radiographer
- **Chapter 13:** The CT Technologists
- **Chapter 14:** Artificial Intelligence on CT Imaging
- **Chapter 15:** AERB Requirements for Installation of CT Scan
- **Chapter 16:** Production of X-rays
- **Chapter 17:** Generations of CT System
- **Chapter 18:** Collimators and Filtration
- **Chapter 19:** Components of CT Scanner
- **Chapter 20:** Hounsfield Scale
- **Chapter 21:** Image Reconstruction
- **Chapter 22:** Window Setting
- **Chapter 23:** Three-Dimensional Imaging
- **Chapter 24:** Volumetric Rendering Techniques
- **Chapter 25:** CT Fluoroscopy
- **Chapter 26:** CT Contrast
- **Chapter 27:** CT Myelography
- **Chapter 28:** CT Angiography
- **Chapter 29:** Artifacts
- **Chapter 30:** Thermoluminescent Dosimeter

Chapter 31: Diagnosis on CT Images
Chapter 32: Interventional Radiology
Chapter 33: Tidbits on CT Scan
Chapter 34: CT Scan versus MRI Scan
Chapter 35: Medical Records
Chapter 36: Radiation Units
Chapter 37: Radiation Hazards
Chapter 38: Radiation Protection
Chapter 39: Picture Archiving and Communication System
Chapter 40: Cloud Computing
Chapter 41: Photon-Counting Detector CT
Chapter 42: CT Technologist Questions/Answers

CHAPTER 12

Radiography and the Radiographer

RADIOGRAPHY

Radiography is a blend of science and art of radiation for formation of images of the tissues and organs of human body.

RADIOGRAPHER

The radiographer is responsible for creation of diagnostic images by accurate positioning, appropriate use of technology and caring for the patient's needs.

With this special ability he contributes and assists in the diagnosis of sickness.

CHAPTER 13

The CT Technologist

RADIOLOGY TECHNOLOGIST

Radiology technologists are trained during their educational program and are fully trained by the time they start their careers. A technologist specializes in using technology and completely understands the technology and other technologies that can be applied.

He determines what can be improved in the industry and how to incorporate new technology, find new ways to resolve problems and tries to further develop various processes.

CT SCAN TECHNOLOGIST

A CT scan technologist has expert-level equipment operation skills. He is responsible for assisting patients and operating equipment to perform examinations. He prepares and calibrates the equipment. He explains the process to the patients, positions them for the scan and helps them remain calm during the procedure. After the procedure, the technologist evaluates the image closely to make sure it's clear.

They Also Achieve

- **Image reconstruction:** They reconstruct images for diagnosis and treatment from the scan.
- **Radiation safety:** CT scans involve the use of ionizing radiation, they have good understanding of radiation safety protocols.
- **CPR, intravenous insertion and other health care skills:** Since a CT scan technologist works in a health care facility with other staff, they have additional medical skills to assist radiologists or other providers as needed.
- **Patient care:** To help patients feel calm and understand the scan procedures, a technologist has strong communication skills, patience and empathy.
- They maintain patients' medical records.
- **Good anatomical knowledge:** The technologist applies knowledge of the human anatomy to recognize abnormalities.

This will be increasing demand for CT technologists as the population ages; more people require CT scans and more diagnostic centers being opened.

CHAPTER 14

Artificial Intelligence on CT Imaging

Artificial intelligence (AI) based deep learning post-processing and reconstruction holds promise on clinical, operational and financial aspect of CT imaging. It has the potential to reduce radiation dose exposure consistently below current industry levels by reducing image noise and improving image quality for all types of CT studies. This results in profound impact on quality, efficiency and cost of imaging procedures, more so in pediatric and lung studies. Where low-dose protocols are in place, AI derived approaches can further improve diagnostic quality, modality utilization and radiology efficiency.

As patients are becoming aware of hazards of radiation, they are seeking programs that can offer the lowest attainable dose. As Low As Reasonably Attainable (ALARA) has new meaning with the use of the new Deep Learning Reconstruction (DLR) and post-processing approaches which give provider a commercial advantage. They will stand out among other providers by offering their patients the safest and most reliable CT screening programs.

Early adopters of DLR and associated AI post-processing technology stand to realize immediate returns in terms of image quality, diagnostic accuracy and technology, with resultant satisfaction, to both the radiologist and the patients.

Longer term improved efficiency and modality utilization have the potential to deliver significant additional advantage in operational and financial performance.

AERB Requirements for Installation of CT Scan

Atomic Energy Regulatory Board (AERB) regulates radiation facilities and activities to ensure that the use of ionizing radiation and nuclear energy in India does not cause undue risk to health and environment.

After satisfactory inspection of site and documentation, AERB issues a license/registration for operation of the radiation equipment.

AERB requirements for installing CT scan, the size of the room housing the gantry of the CT unit shall not be less than 25 m². More than one unit of any type of radiation shall not be installed in the same room.

AERB license for Medical Diagnostic X-ray equipment ensures that equipment meets the quality requirements. AERB has standardized requisite Quality Assurance (QA) tests requirements to ensure that acceptable diagnostic image is obtainable with optimal radiation dose to patient.

The effective dose (exposure) per CT scan at 1 meter will not exceed 15 μSv (1.6 mR) in any direction. The radiation dose to the members of public living nearby shall not exceed annual limit of 1 mSv (i.e., 1000 microsieverts).

For CT equipments, in addition to Operator and Medical Practitioner, Radiological Safety Officer (RSO) is mandatory.

Once the license is issued, it is valid for 5 years. Before expiry of the license, it needs to be renewed by providing necessary details as specified by AERB. AERB does not charge any fees for issuance of license/registration for operation of any radiation equipment.

The effective doses from diagnostic CT procedures are typically estimated to be in the range of 1 to 5 mSv. To reduce radiation exposure one must remember the 3 principles—time, distance, and shielding.

CHAPTER 16

Production of X-rays

CT scan uses X-rays to produce images, the technology used to produce X-rays in conventional X-ray equipment and CT equipment is the same.

X-rays are invisible, highly penetrating, electromagnetic radiations having wavelength of 0.1-1 Å (Armstrong) in the range of 0.01 to 10 nanometers and speed is same as that of light (3 x 108 m/sec). They are considered as a form of modified electrons. X-ray tube is a diode consisting of tungsten filament cathode and a rotating anode target of tungsten held in an evacuated glass.

Tungsten anode is inclined at an angle so that it works on line-focus principle. X-rays are produced when the electron beam strikes the anode made of tungsten or molybdenum. Tungsten (atomic number 74) is used as target material for X-ray production. Molybdenum (atomic number 42) is used as the target in mammography. Cathode is connected to the negative terminal and consists of small coil of wire made of tungsten (filament). Cathode generates the electrons from the electric circuit and focuses them into well-defined beam aimed at anode. Anode is relatively large piece of metal that connects to positive end of electric circuit. It converts electronic energy into X-rays and rapidly dissipates heat produced during this process. Anode is made up of tungsten because it has high melting point, low rate of evaporation and maintains strength at high temperature **(Fig. 1)**.

The electrons are produced by cathode filament by electric current, emitting photoelectrons. The electrons coming from the filament cathode are then accelerated towards the target anode by a large electrical potential applied between the filament and target. When the beam of electrons hits the target anode there is rapid deceleration of electrons leading to emission of X-rays and heat. About 1% of the energy generated is emitted as X-rays. The rest of the energy

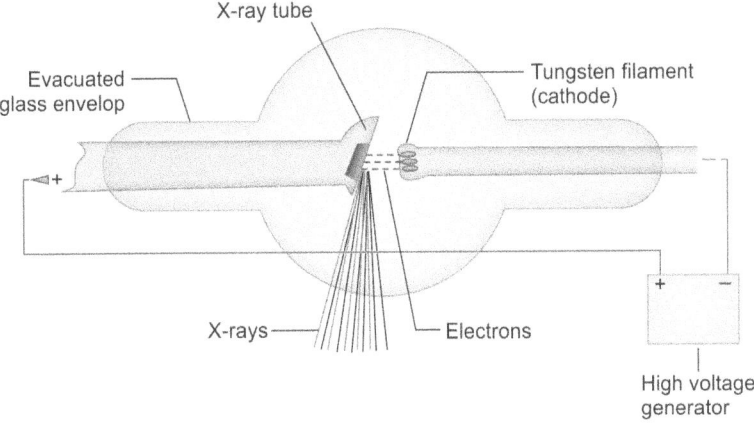

Fig. 1: Line diagram showing production of X-rays.

is released as heat. The assembly of cathode and anode is enclosed in an envelope which is made of glass. It provides support and electric insulation, keeps cathode and anode in air tight enclosure and maintains vacuum in tube.

Housing is the outermost covering that encloses and supports the envelope. It is filled with oil that provides electric insulation, allows heat dissipation and cooling. Modern X-ray tubes are based on hot cathode tube principle invented by Coolidge in 1913 which enables excellent control of kVp (kilovolt peak) and mAs (milliampere second). kVp is responsible for penetration of X-ray beam, low kVp gives high contrast. mAs is responsible for the film blackening. The radiation intensity on the cathode side of the X-ray tube is higher than on the anode side and this principle is called as the **heel effect**. The heat generated in the tube is dissipated in three ways—conduction, convection and radiation. Diagnostic X-ray machine uses voltage up to 150 kVp whereas machines used for radiotherapy use high voltage >200 kV.

Two different interactions give rise to X-rays. Interactions with electron shell produce characteristic X-rays photons, while interaction with atomic nucleus produces bremsstrahlung X-ray photons. In diagnostic radiology about 85% of X-rays arise from bremsstrahlung radiation and 15% from characteristic radiation. X-ray filter made of aluminium absorbs low energy radiation and decreases unnecessary patient exposure and thus improves film contrast. Grid is made of parallel lead lines with intervening radiolucent material. It absorbs scattered radiation. Cones and collimators restrict field size and decrease scatter. Distance from X-ray tube (focus) to the X-ray film is called focus film distance (FFD). It is 100 cm for usual radiographs of extremities, abdomen and skull. However, for standing radiograph of chest it is 180 cm (6 ft) so as to reduce the magnification.

CHAPTER 17

Generations of CT System

CT scan after its introduction in 1971 with a single detector for brain study by Sir Godfrey Hounsfield, scanner has undergone multiple improvements with an increase in the number of detectors and a decrease in the scan time. CT generations are depicted in **Table 1**.

Table 1: The CT generations for understanding the geometric differences.

Generations	Years	Developed	Region	Movement of Detector	Time to Acquire Image	Why Obsolete?
1st	1971	To show CT works	Head only	Translate-Rotate	~5 min	Slow
2nd	1974	Image faster	Head only	Translate-Rotate	20 sec–2 min	Slow
3rd	1975	Image faster	All anatomy	Rotate-Rotate	1 sec	
4th	1976	Make images without rings	All anatomy	Rotate-Stationary	1 sec	Expensive, not good for scatter
5th	1980	Fast cardiac CT	Cardiac only	Stationary-Stationary	50 ms	Cardiac specific, low X-ray flux

FIRST GENERATION CT SYSTEM (ROTATE-TRANSLATE, PENCIL BEAM)

The first generation CT scanners were designed to acquire CT images of the patient's head and were based on parallel-beam geometry with translate-rotate principle of tube and detector combination **(Fig. 1)**. These scanners used a thin slit X-ray beam and single X-ray detector to acquire the entire CT image. The X-ray head and detector were mounted on a C-arm frame and onto a synchronized linear scan mechanism that could be rotated through an arc of 180°. The C-arm would be rotated into position stopped and held still while the linear scanning mechanism moved the thin slit X-ray beam across the anatomical view. Small detector monitored the intensity of beam before entering body to yield value of incident intensity. Each linear scan produced one view or X-ray image. The C-arm would be positioned in 1° steps to allow 180 linear scans along the 180° arc. The linear scan mechanism allowed 240 detector measurements at 1.7 mm intervals to create each of the 180 views. Some scanners had two X-ray beams and a second detector to allow the scanner to acquire two anatomical section scans at the same time. A complete CT scan and image reconstruction took upto 10 minutes. The disadvantages were long scanning time and compromised image quality due to patient motion.

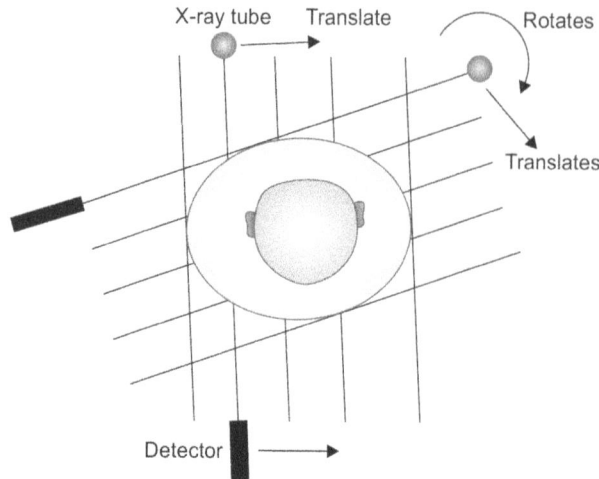

Fig. 1: First generation CT system with linear scan of source and detector—rotate/translate, pencil beam scan.

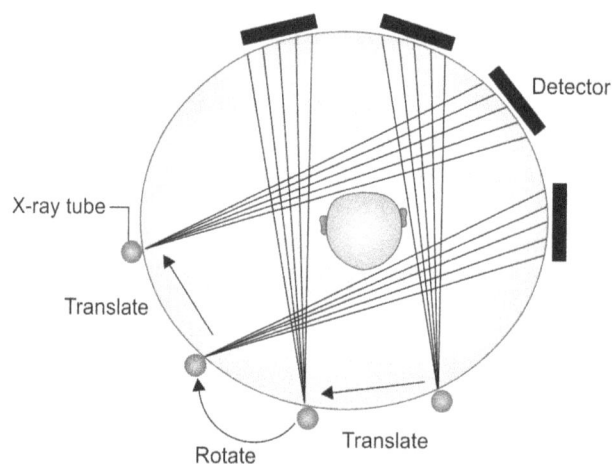

Fig. 2: Second generation CT system—rotate/translate, narrow fan beam with X-ray head and detectors mounted onto-arm frame that could rotate 180°.

SECOND GENERATION SYSTEM (ROTATE-TRANSLATE, NARROW FAN BEAM)

A fan-shaped X-ray beam (3–10° diverging angle) was projected onto a linear array of approximately 30 detectors. The X-ray head and detectors were mounted onto a C-arm frame that could rotate 180° around the patient **(Fig. 2)**. The increased number of detectors reduced the number of linear scans required during the 180° arc, reducing the time required for a scan to less than 90 seconds. Reduced scan times allowed the patient to hold their breath for the entire scan allowing the radiographer to scan the thoracic region of the body. The fan-shaped beam increased scatter radiation artifact forcing the use of lead masks on the detectors to reduce this scatter radiation artifact.

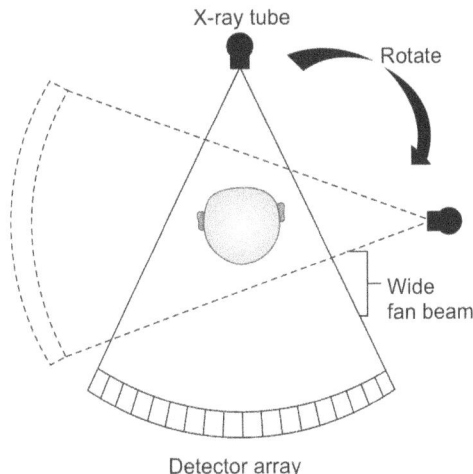

Fig. 3: Third generation CT system—rotate-rotate, wide fan beam—An arc of detectors and X-ray tube rotate continuously around patient for 360°.

THIRD GENERATION SYSTEM (ROTATE-ROTATE, WIDE FAN BEAM)

A wider fan-shaped X-ray beam (50 to 55°) and a curved array of 250 to 750 detectors **(Fig. 3)**. The wider beam and larger detector array allowed the scanner to include the entire body in a single exposure. An arc of detectors and X-ray tube rotate continuously around patient for 360° eliminating the need for linear scanning to be combined with the X-ray head rotation **(Fig. 3)**. Third generation scanners would acquire approximately 700,000 measurements per anatomical section. Scan times reduced to less than 12 seconds. Shorter scan times allowed sequential scans to approximated dynamic functions with approximately 4 scans per minute. In this configuration, detectors are fixed radially and do not view scan areas uniformly with only center detectors in arc, see the pixels at center of field of view (FOV). However, this fixed relationship allows detectors to be highly collimated reducing scatter radiation and hence image noise. Spatial resolution, a key image parameter of CT depends on how closely spaced are detectors (number of detectors in an arc). Number of detectors in arc ranges from 600 to more than 900, limiting spatial resolution to 5-to-10 line pairs per centimeter. However, the single detector array made third generation scanners prone to ring artifact.

FOURTH GENERATION SYSTEM (ROTATE-STATIONARY)

A single projection wide angle fan-shaped X-ray beam (50 to 55°) and fixed detector arc with 600 to 2000 stationary detectors. The detectors are fixed in a circular ring around the patient and X-ray head and alignment of the X-ray beam to each detector is essential **(Fig. 4)**. The X-ray head travels more than 360° in order to provide an acceleration and deceleration zone. Scanning takes place as the X-ray head travels in either direction, clockwise and counterclockwise. Scan rates of approximately 15 scans per minute are achieved and are limited by the interscan time used to change the direction of the X-ray head travel. Dynamic scanning and overscanning modes using scanning arcs of greater than 360° are available. This geometry permits very high spatial resolution (more than 20 lines/cm). However, there is increased detection of scattered radiation leading to image noise.

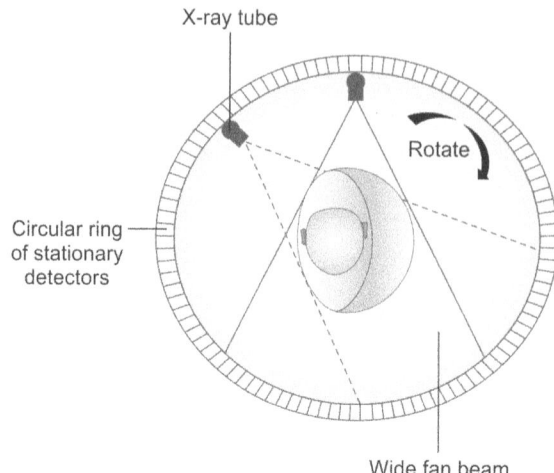

Fig. 4: Fourth generation system (rotate/stationary)—detectors are fixed in circular ring around the patient and X-ray head which travels more than 360°.

FIFTH GENERATION

Stationary-stationary, electron beam: A novel CT scanner was developed for cardiac tomographic imaging. This "cine CT" scanner does not use a conventional X-ray tube and is usually used in cardiology. A large ring that circles the patients is used which lies directly opposed to the detector ring. The X-rays are produced from the focal track as a high energy electron beam. There are no moving parts to this scanner gantry. The electron beam is produced in a vacuum pump. It is capable of 50-milisecond scan times and can produce 17 CT slices each second for example in heart structures.

VOLUME (SPIRAL/HELICAL) CT

Spiral CT design makes it possible to achieve greater rotational velocities than conventional systems, which allows for shorter scan time. The aim of spiral CT is to obtain meaningful CT data as patient move through rotating, continuous fan beam exposure. Instead of obtaining data sequentially during individual exposure; a block of data in the form of corkscrew or helix is obtained **(Fig. 5)**. If the table movement occurs at such a speed that during one revolution of tube patient is moved by distance equal to slice thickness complete volume of tissue is examined. Before advent of spiral CT, in third and fourth generation CT data is obtained in discrete slices of patient anatomy in a method commonly called axial scanning. In axial scanning, each revolution of X-ray tube around patient produces single data set (slice). During data collection patient table is motionless. To create an additional slice, table is advanced to given amount and X-ray tube is once again rotated around the patient.

Advanced slip ring technology is used to allow the X-ray head to travel in one direction indefinitely. The X-ray head does not have to be decelerated and accelerated in between scans. Approximately 1000 detectors are aligned opposite the X-ray tube. The moving detector array travels in a circle around the patient at the same time as the X-ray head moves. The patient can be advanced through the CT gantry as the continuously revolving X-ray head circles the patient **(Fig. 5)**. The computer acquires measurements from the detectors that result in data representing a continuous helical scan. The primary advantage to helical scans is the reduced scan time for example the entire abdomen can be scanned in single breath hold. This results

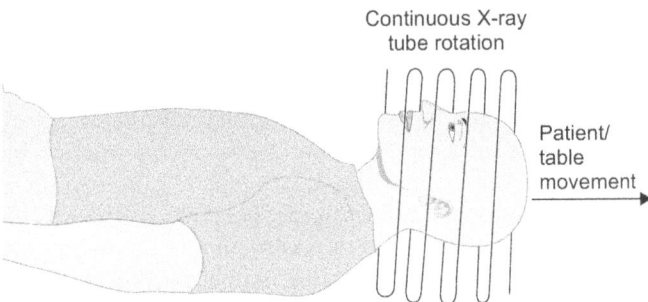

Fig. 5: Volume (spiral/helical) CT—X-ray tube rotates continuously and the patient moves through the X-ray beam at a constant rate.

in the use of less contrast media and less motion artifact. The primary disadvantage is that the entire 360° scan information is not acquired for every anatomical cross section. Computer reconstruction is required to fill in the missing data. Three key advances enable CT data to be acquired continuously with ongoing patient movement—slip-ring technology, precise patient table transport and software reconstruction algorithms.

SLIP-RING TECHNOLOGY

In conventional CT systems, there was inherent delay of 3 to 5 seconds between each exposure which arose from physical need to have cables connecting stationary gantry and rotating tube-detector assembly. After 1 to 3 exposure, depending on cable length, the cable become wound and then rotation of tube-detector assembly had to stop, change direction to unwind. Slip-ring technology abolished the physical need for presence of electric cable between generator and moving tube-detector assembly. In this, power from generator is connected to large stationary ring and other large ring that house the X-ray-detector assembly moves around within stationary ring. Power is transmitted between stationary and moving ring by means of brushes making it possible to have continuous X-ray tube rotation (rather than back and forth) and continuous data acquisition.

MULTISLICE SPIRAL CT

All multislice spiral CT system use third generation geometry with added dimension of multiple arcs of detectors. The first deployment of this technology include dual-arc detector in which two parallel arcs of detectors are used to simultaneously acquire data during single revolution of scan frame dividing total X-ray beam into two equal beams.

ANALOG-TO-DIGITAL CONVERSION OF SIGNAL

Once the detector generates the analog or electrical signal it is directed to the data acquisition system (DAS). The analog signal generated by the detector is a weak signal and must be amplified to be further analyzed which is done by the data acquisition system (DAS). The DAS is located in the gantry right after or above the detector system, however, in some modern CT scans the signal amplification occurs within the detector itself. The projection of raw data is in the form of an electrical or analog signal, which is first converted to digital information before sending to the computer. This task is accomplished by an analog to digital converter which is an essential component of the DAS. The digital signal is transferred to an array processor which solve the statistical information using algorithmic calculations essential for mathematical reconstruction of a CT image. Reconstruction is conversion of digital data provided by data acquisition system to a form image that is suitable for viewing on the monitor. An array processor is a specialized high-speed computer designed to execute mathematical algorithms for the purpose of reconstruction and solves reconstruction mathematics faster than a standard microprocessor. Special algorithms may require several seconds to several minutes for a standard microprocessor to compute. Recently, processors termed as image or reconstruction generator that compute CT reconstruction mathematics faster than an array processor has been utilized to solve reconstruction mathematics essential to the development of CT fluoroscopy.

For each ray projection measurement made during CT scan, fundamental equation ($I = I_0 e_{-mx}$) is generated and complete set of such equations must then be solved to obtain individual value of 'm' for each matrix element by the computer system. Many methods have been devised to solve set of equations generated in scan of which commonly used is *filtered back-projection* method. To eliminate blurring filtering or convolution "kernel" is used. Two types of filters or kernels used are—smooth (low frequency) filter to examine soft tissue and edge enhancement (high frequency) filter to examine bone.

CHAPTER 18

Collimators and Filtration

CT systems feature various collimators, filters and shielding designs, which provide filtration of the X-ray spectra, definition of the measured slices, guarding detectors against scattered radiation and general radiation protection. These vary from scan to scan but always offer the same functions.

COLLIMATION

Collimation in CT serves to ensure good image quality and to reduce unnecessary radiation doses for the patient.

Collimators are present between the X-ray source and the patient (tube or pre-patient collimators) and between the patient and the detectors (detector or post-patient collimators).

The tube collimator is used to shape the X-ray fan beam before it penetrates the patient (restrict the X-ray flux applied to a narrow region defines the shape of the X-ray beam). It consists of a set of collimator blades made of highly absorbing materials such as tungsten or molybdenum. The opening of these blades is adjusted according to the selected slice width and the size and position of the focal spot. It defines slice thickness for single-slice CT. Tube collimators define the dose profile according to the required slice thickness. Post-patient collimators improve the slice sensitivity profile by giving a more rectangular shape.

FILTRATION

The X-ray photons emitted by the X-ray tube exhibit a wide spectrum. The soft, low-energy X-rays, which contribute strongly to the patient dose and scatter radiation but less to the detected signal are removed. To achieve this goal, most CT manufacturers use X-ray filters.

The inherent filtration of the X-ray-tube, typically 3 mm aluminium equivalent thickness, is the first filter. In addition, flat or shaped filters can be used. Flat filters, made of copper or aluminium, are placed between the X-ray source and the patient. They modify the X-ray spectrum uniformly across the entire field of view. Because the cross-section of a patient is mostly oval-shaped, some manufacturers use shaped (or bow-tie) filter. These filters have an increased thickness from center to periphery, allowing them to attenuate radiation, hardly at all in the center but strongly in the periphery. They are made from a material with a low atomic number and high density such as Teflon.

In some machines comb-shaped collimators close to the detector array are used to decrease the effective detector element width and thus increase the achievable geometrical resolution.

CHAPTER 19

Components of CT Scanner

In CT two-dimensional pictures represent three-dimensional human body. The images are produced by converting electrical energy to X-ray photons, the X-ray photons pass through 360° at a point. The density of the different parts of the body changes the intensity of photons passing through it. The computer processes the differences in transmitted X-ray photon numbers to produce data that recreates and displays sequential images as 2D CT sections on the monitor which can be converted to CT film.

CT scan combines a series of X-ray images taken from different angles around the body and uses computer processing to create cross-sectional images (slices) showing tissues inside the body, at the level of the section. CT scan unit depicted in **Figure 1.**

CT SCANNING HARDWARE (FIG. 2)

- ❖ Generator
- ❖ Scanning unit (gantry)
    - ◆ X-ray tubes
    - ◆ Photon detectors
    - ◆ X-rays shielding elements
- ❖ Patient table
- ❖ Image processor
- ❖ Console (control unit)

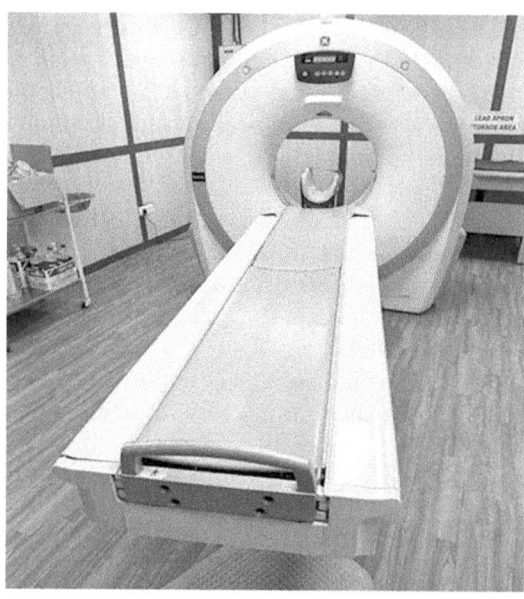

Fig. 1: CT scan unit.

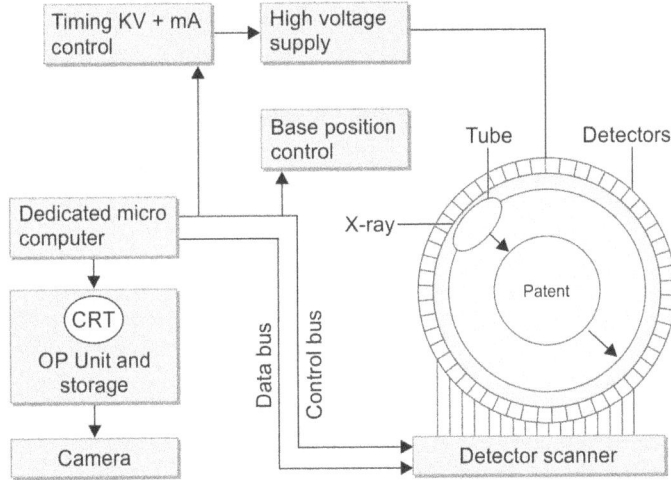

Fig. 2: Line diagram of CT unit.

X-RAY GENERATOR

CT scanners today use high frequency generators to produce X-ray required for CT protocols. The operating frequency ranges from 5 to 50 kHz and generator power can range from 15 to 60 KW which supports exposure technique from 80 to 140 kV and 30 to 500 mA.

Slip ring technology eliminated the need for cables and allows continuous rotation of the gantry components without interference of cables.

THE SCANNING UNIT (GANTRY)

Gantry is the scanning unit. It contains the X-ray tube with shielding and photon detectors. The X-ray tube and photon detectors are positioned opposite each other and are made to rotate 360° in one direction around the patient.

The gantry tilt is the angle formed between the X-ray tube plane and the vertical plane in modern machines, gantry tilt ranges between -25 degrees and +25 degrees.

The use of slip rings in gantries allows continuous complete circular movements of the internal elements without the internal circuits and cables becoming entangled. The gantry contains round opening with diameter of 60-85 cm for the table and the patient to pass through.

X-ray Tube

The X-ray tube converts moving electrons into X-ray photons. The X-ray tube is composed of a cathode assembly, an anode assembly, and a rotor, all contained in a tube envelope and together called the tube insert. The air/gas inside the tube envelope is evacuated, forming a vacuum.

The X-ray tube cathode filament is made of tungsten, it expels the electrons by thermionic emission. The current from the X-ray generator passing through the filament boils off electrons. The emitted electrons are accelerated by the potential difference between the cathode and anode toward the tungsten anode.

The X-ray tube needs the design which will absorb high heat levels generated from the high-speed rotation of the anode and the bombardment of electrons upon the anode surface. An X-ray tubes heat capacity is expressed in heat units. Modern CT systems utilize X-ray tubes that have a heat capacity of approximately 2 to 7 million heat units (MHU) with cooling rates as fast as 1 mhu/min. CT X-ray tubes utilize a combination of oil and air-cooling systems to eliminate heat and maintain continuous operation.

CT tubes utilize a bigger filament than conventional radiography X-ray tubes which increases the size of the effective focal spot. Decreasing the anode or target angle decreases the size of the effective focal spot.

The anode angle of a conventional radiography tube is between 7° and 10°. In CT, this angle is decreased to help alleviate some of the effects caused by the heel effect.

Photon Detectors

Detectors collect information regarding the degree to which each anatomic structure attenuated the beam during the exposure. Instead of film to record, the attenuated beam digital X-ray detectors collect the information.

The two basic detector types used in CT are scintillation (solid-state) and ionization (xenon gas) detectors. Current detectors use scintillation (solid-state) detectors.

Individual detector elements are affixed to a circuit board. Solid state crystal detectors are made from a variety of materials, such as cadmium tungstate, cesium iodide, bismuth germanate and ceramic rare earth compounds like gadolinium or yttrium.

Now all scanners are multi-slice and have 8-64 or more rows of detectors. There are generally 1000-2000 detectors

When the X-ray beam travels through the patient, it is attenuated by the anatomical structures it passes through. The CT process relies on collecting attenuated photon energy and converting it to an electrical signal, which is then converted to a digital signal for computer reconstruction. A detector is a crystal that when struck by an X-ray photon produces light or electrical energy.

The two types of detectors utilized in CT systems are scintillation or solid state and xenon gas detectors. Scintillation detectors utilize a crystal that fluoresces when struck by an X-ray photon which produces light energy. A photodiode which transforms the light energy into electrical or analog energy is attached to the scintillation portion of the detector. The strength of the detector signal is proportional to the number of attenuated photons that are successfully converted to light energy and then to an electrical or analog signal.

The signal represents an absorption or attenuation profile which is obtained for each view or projection and every detector in the detector array is responsible for this task. The most frequently used scintillation crystals are made of bismuth germanate and cadmium tungstate.

It is important that detectors are placed as close to one another as possible. Scintillation detectors convert 99 to 100% of the attenuated photons into a useable electrical signal.

X-Ray Shielding Elements

X-rays that do not travel in a straight path from the X-ray tube to the detector that is in line with the beam but instead reach an off-path, detector lead to reconstruct an accurate representation of what signal was derived from original location. Phenomenons and inaccuracies in image processing, result in image "noise," which reduces the contrast between imaged structures that is a critical element for maintaining image quality and enabling interpretation of the anatomy and pathology.

PATIENT TABLE

The patient's table moves through the gantry during the scan. The distance of table moves during a complete rotation of the gantry is referred to as the table pitch or detector pitch. Table pitch equals the forward table movement in millimeters during a complete gantry rotation divided by beam collimation (the slice thickness in mm). Faster moving tables are described as having greater pitches. Increased table speed reduces scanning time and radiation dose but reduces image resolution if the circuitry of the machine cannot process the information as quickly as the table moves.

IMAGE PROCESSOR

The formation of a CT image is a distinct three phases process. The scanning phase produces data, but not an image. The reconstruction phase processes the acquired data and forms a digital image. The visible and displayed analog image (shades of gray) is produced by the digital-to analog conversion phase.

CT scan combines a series of X-ray images taken from different angles around your body and uses computer processing to create cross-sectional images (slices) of the bones, blood vessels and soft tissues inside the body. The digital signal is stored as bits and bytes on the processor chip as data that contains information about the scan. This data can be manipulated using mathematical algorithms to represent the 3D structure in different ways as different types of images. In general, formulas are applied to convert the data from its original reference values to new values, referred to as "transformation."

Images are displayed on monitor screen. Monitor screens are composed pixels. Each pixel represents a two-dimensional projection of a three-dimensional volume, which is termed a voxel. Each voxel and pixel are assigned a Hounsfield number reflecting the amount of photon energy absorbed and measured by the detector, which reflects the density of the object at the time of the scan. The larger the number, the greater the brightness of the displayed pixel.

CONSOLE

Often there are two different control consoles, one used by the CT scan operator, and the other used by the radiologist.

CHAPTER 20

Hounsfield Scale

Hounsfield scale or unit (HU) **(Fig. 1)** was crafted Hounsfield a dimensionless quantity used to express a linear transformation of the measured attenuation coefficient (radiodensity) in the form of a simple number. In the early stage of CT, radiologists would use large paper printouts of Hounsfield units to interpret brain scans.

Radiodensity on CT is measured in Hounsfield Units (HU). HU range from -1000 to +3000. By definition water or CSF = 0. Air is (-)1000 because it is the least dense structure. Bone is the densest and measures +1000. Fat is less dense than water and therefore measures (-)100. Brain parenchyma is denser than water and ranges from +20 to +40. White matter is less dense than gray matter due to the fat within the myelin within the white matter. Acute blood is bright on CT and measures + 55 to +75 HU. Calcification is denser than blood and will measure in the low 100–300 HU. Very dense bone may show upto +2000 HU eg cochlea and over 3000 HU for metals.

The software of all CT scanners and picture archiving and communications systems (PACS) have the ability to measure the density of a region of interest (ROI) electronically overlaid the image.

Hounsfield units are measured and reported in a variety of clinical applications. One well-known use is the evaluation of the fat content of the liver, with fatty liver diagnosed by the presence of a liver-to-spleen ratio <1.0 or 0.8, provide definitive diagnosis in lipomas anywhere in the body.

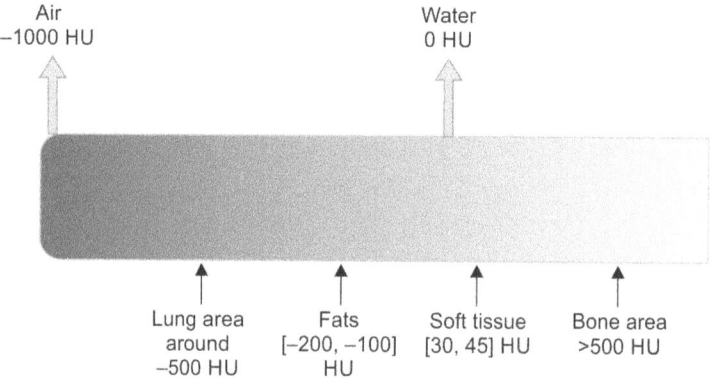

Fig. 1: Shows different structures on CT with their relative HU values.

CT NUMBER SCALE

CT number is linear attenuation coefficient of X-rays, is given by:
CT number = K (M-Mw) Mw
Where,
Mw-attenuation coefficient of water
M-attenuation coefficient of pixel in question
K-1000 (original EMI scanner used value of 500)
In honor of Godfrey Hounsfield, CT unit is called a *Hounsfield unit (HU)*. Air has value of (–)1000 *HU*, water 0 *HU*, bone +1000 *HU*.

Image Reconstruction

CHAPTER 21

The acquisition of volumetric data using spiral CT means that the images can be postprocessed in ways appropriate to the clinical situation.

Multiplanar reformatting (MPR) is by taking standard axial images and subject to the three-dimensional array of CT numbers obtained with a series of contiguous slices; and can be viewed in sagittal, coronal, oblique and paraxial planes **(Figs. 1A to C)**.

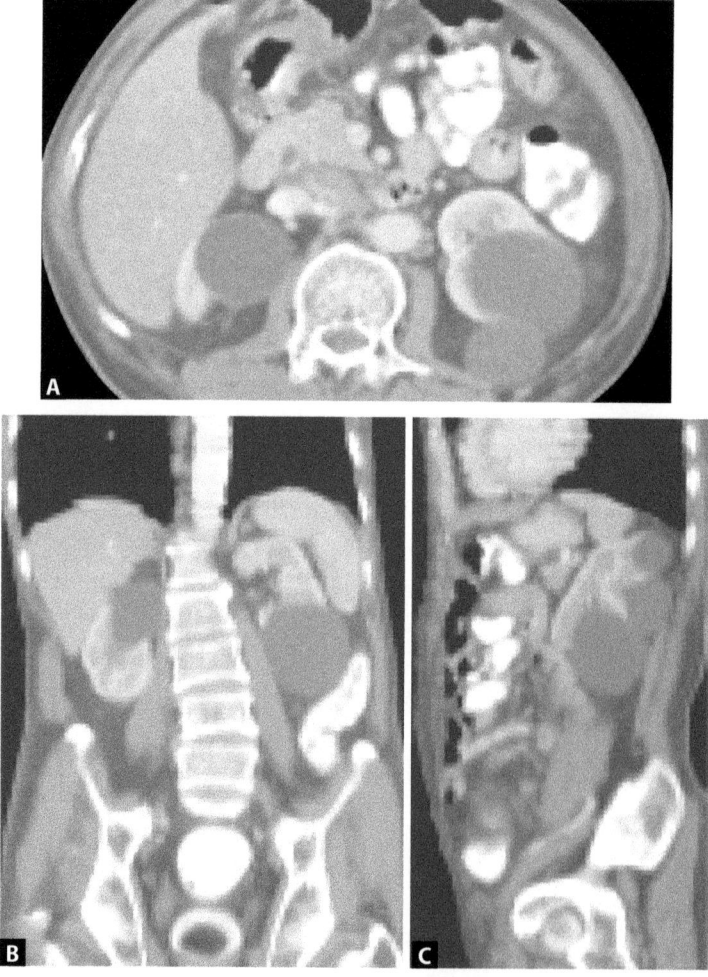

Figs. 1A to C: Bilateral renal cysts seen in axial section: (A) Reformatted into; (B) Coronal; (C) Sagittal planes.

CHAPTER 22

Window Setting

The meaning or full form of WINDOWS is Wide Interactive Network Development for Office Work Solution.

Windowing or image enhancement is the process in which the CT image is manipulated by CT numbers, to change the appearance of the picture and highlight particular structures. The contrast is adjusted via the window width. The brightness of the image is adjusted via the window level.

WINDOW WIDTH

The window width is the measure of the range of CT numbers that an image contains. A wider window width (2000 HU), therefore, will display a wider range of CT numbers. Consequently, the transition of dark to light structures will occur over a larger transition area to that of a narrow window width (<1000 HU).

A wide window displaying all the CT numbers will result in different attenuations between soft tissues to become obscured.

Wide window: Wide window (W) is 400-2000 HU best used in areas of acute differing attenuation values; a good example is lungs or cortical tissue, where air and vessels will sit side by side.

Narrow window: Narrow window is 50-350 HU are excellent when examining areas of similar attenuation, for example, soft tissues.

WINDOW LEVEL

The window level (WL) or (W) or window center is the midpoint of the range of the CT numbers displayed.

When the window level is decreased the CT image will be brighter and if window level is increased the CT image will appear dark.

Below are the width (W) and level (L) generally used (the values are in Hounsfield Units - HU):

- **Head and neck**
  - Brain—W: 80 L: 40
  - Subdural—W: 130-300 L: 50-100
  - Temporal bones—W: 2800 L: 600 or W: 4000 L: 700
  - Soft tissues—W: 350-400 L: 20-60
- **Chest**
  - Lungs—W: 1500 L: 600
  - Mediastinum—W: 350 L: 50
- **Abdomen**
  - Soft tissues—W: 400 L:50
  - Liver—W: 150 L: 30

- **Spine**
  - Soft tissues—W: 250 L: 50
  - Bone—W: 1800 L: 400

Adjustment of what is visible in the image based on adjusting the visible HU. This is referred to as "windowing" or "changing the window." The window width determines image contrast. The greater the width, the less is the contrast. Window width represents the range of HU included in the image.

CHAPTER 23

Three-Dimensional Imaging

Many fractures of the mandible associated with frontal bone with or without walls of sinuses can be reconstructed into a 3-dimensional image **(Figs. 1A to D)**.

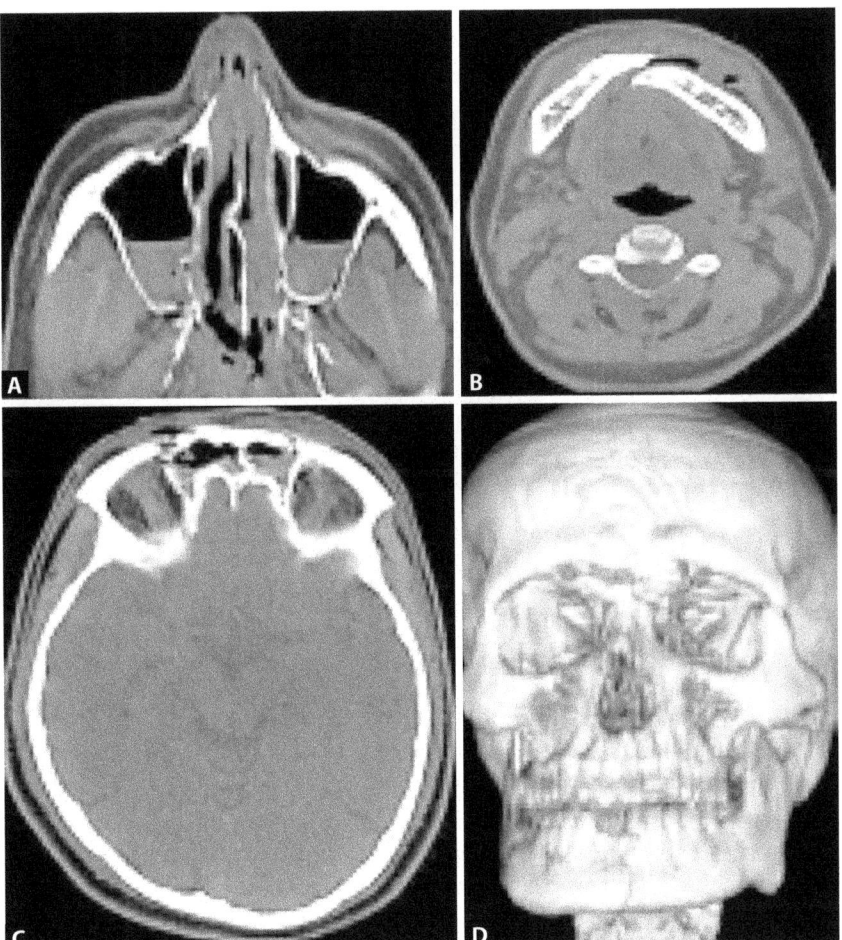

Figs. 1A to D: (A to C) Fracture of body of mandible and frontal bone with bilateral maxillary hemosinus; (D) 3D image of face including mandible.

CHAPTER 24

Volumetric Rendering Techniques

CT volumetric rendering techniques include maximum intensity projection—MIP, minimum intensity projection—MinIP, shaded surface display—SSD, volume rendering—VR and virtual endoscopy provide increased diagnostic potential.

MAXIMUM INTENSITY PROJECTION

Maximum intensity projection (MIP) displays voxels with the highest density (HU) on every view through the 3D image volume. MIPs display high-density structures, such as bone and contrast-filled arteries, better than SSD. MIPs are used for CT arteriography for detecting emboli in the pulmonary arteries. The MIP algorithm is diagnostically useful because it can readily distinguish structures that are hyperdense with respect to surrounding tissues.

Detecting voxels with higher density enables the radiologist to better understand the extension and morphology of some structures, such as vessels, nodules, calcifications, surgical clips, foreign bodies, etc., and significantly reduces the time needed to analyze complex structures in different planes and with a non-linear course. This method is particularly useful in daily practice to detect small lung nodules.

MIP is also used in angiography because it can detect the opacity of a vessel against tissues with lower densities and, therefore, can follow the complete course of the structures containing contrast agents even if they are tortuous, as is the case with gastric varicose veins. In particular, it is possible to acquire various MIP images, each one obtained from a slightly more angulated point of view with respect to the preceding one so that the perception of rotation is created; this is especially useful for the analysis of complex vascular structures.

MINIMUM INTENSITY PROJECTION

Minimum-intensity projection (MinIP) displays voxels with the lowest density. MinIP is suitable to highlight air-filled structures, such as the bronchial tree.

MinIP is a data visualization method that enables detection of low-density structures in a given volume. The algorithm uses all the data in a volume of interest to generate a single bidimensional image. The MinIP algorithm is almost identical to the MIP algorithm but, in the case of MinIP, for each XY coordinate only the lowest Hounsfield value along the Z axis is represented. In this way, only the most hypodense structures of the volume are represented, regardless of their plane of location. For example, by performing a MinIP mapping of the thorax before administration of contrast, an image of the bronchial tree can be generated since the bronchi, being air-filled, are the least dense structures of the thorax.

MinIP algorithm is particularly useful for analyzing the bile tree and pancreatic duct, which are hypodense compared to surrounding tissue, especially in the pancreatic and portal phase of contrast agent administration.

SHADED SURFACE DISPLAY

Shaded surface display (SSD) or surface rendering, selects voxels to display based on a selected range of HU. SSD includes or excludes voxels from the image based on algorithms set to detect differences in density at the edge of structures where surfaces have different densities.

SHADED SURFACE DISPLAY VOLUME RENDERING TECHNIQUE

Shaded surface display volume rendering technique (SS-VRT) creates a 3D visual illustration of CT volumetric data for display from any desired perspective. SS-VRT images provide a sensation of three-dimensionality that is significantly superior to other volume rendering techniques. The SS-VRT techniques are quite complex and processor intensive but are now becoming common place. These techniques typically select voxels to be included in a surface rendering based on a selected range of Hounsfield values. By properly choosing the Hounsfield range, different types of tissues can be selected—parenchyma, bone, airways, and vessels. By analyzing a combination of Hounsfield ranges, a volume of CT data can be segmented into several of these tissue types. These techniques then calculate the location of surfaces separating tissue types.

SS-VRT is particularly apt for studying fine details such as articular bone surfaces. The principle diagnostic utility of SS-VRT technique is its ability to represent with great detail structures of a specific density.

However, the potential of these surface modeling techniques is by no means limited to diagnosing small hidden fracture lines. They also are of great use in documenting more extensive lesions, such as multiple rib fractures or complex fractures with multiple dislocated fragments as may be seen in maxillofacial trauma or even distal limb fractures.

VIRTUAL ENDOSCOPY

A particularly important application of surface rendering techniques in CT is virtual endoscopy. The surface rendering technique can be used to simulate an endoscopic exam by locating a point of view inside a hollow organ lumen. When compared to traditional endoscopy, virtual endoscopy has the advantage of being noninvasive and capable of virtually exploring regions inaccessible to an endoscopic device, such as areas distal to a lumen obstruction. Currently, virtual endoscopy has been successfully used for studying a great number of anatomical locations, the most common being the colon, respiratory tract, auditory canal, and urinary tract.

Three-dimensional SSD has also been proposed for assessing the biliary tree. CT cholangiography is possible using an appropriate contrast agent specific for the biliary tract. With proper segmentation, SSD-VR can then be used to perform virtual cholangiography.

CURVED PLANE RECONSTRUCTIONS

Curved plane reconstructions (also called, curved multiplanar reconstructions or curved MPR) are a subcategory of multiplanar reconstructions; instead of representing a plane oriented in one specific direction, they display all voxels contained in a user-selectable curved surface as a single bidimensional image. This allows the user to follow winding structures in their entirety along their natural path of development in a single image. This technique is particularly apt for the study of the vascular system. It is used to display a winding vessel as a straight line and thereby facilitates the identification of vascular defects, stenosis, and dilatations.

However, the field of CT reconstruction techniques is in continuous evolution and newer, even more sophisticated techniques, currently restricted to the research environment, are likely to emerge as technology and diagnostic workstations evolve.

A basic knowledge of these rendering techniques and an appreciation of how they can fit into clinical practice, as well as an idea of how the final images are reconstructed from the original data, are nowadays mandatory skills for every technician and professional working with CT scan images.

CHAPTER 25

CT Fluoroscopy

These two modalities, CT scan and fluoroscopy are combined into a technique called fluoroscopic CT. Around 1995, CT fluoroscopy became popular for viewing live images of the body, like an X-ray movie.

CT scan images offer cross-sectional imaging of the target and its surrounding structures, whereas fluoroscopy offers real-time, imaging, tracking any movement of the target, and its reaction to the biopsy needle.

CT fluoroscopy combines the cross-sectional image targeting provided by CT with the real-time imaging, tracking and movement perception of fluoroscopy for interventional procedures. It allows continuous update of images at a fixed position and is used for CT-guided biopsies and fluid drainages.

CHAPTER 26

CT Contrast

Contrast media when introduced into the body make certain structures or tissues in the body appear different on the images than they would if no contrast material had been administered. Contrast materials help distinguish "contrast" selected areas of the body from surrounding tissue. This helps physicians diagnose medical conditions by improving the visibility of specific organs, blood vessels, or tissues.

Contrast media enter the body in one of several ways. They can be:
- Swallowed (taken by mouth or orally)
- Administered by enema (given rectally)
- Injected into a blood vessel (vein or artery; also referred to as being given intravenously or intra-arterially)
- Injected into spaces within the body.

IODINATED INTRAVASCULAR AGENTS

Intravascular radiological contrast media are iodine containing chemicals which add to the details from any given CT scan study and thereby aid in the diagnosis. They were first introduced by Moses Swick. Iodine (atomic weight 127) is an ideal choice element for X-ray absorption because the korn (K) shell binding energy of iodine (33.7) is nearest to the mean energy used in diagnostic radiography and thus maximum photoelectric interactions can be obtained which are a must for best image quality. These compounds after intravascular injection are rapidly distributed by capillary permeability into extravascular-extracellular space and almost 90% is excreted via glomerular filtration by kidneys within 12 hours.

Following iodinated contrast media are available:
- Ionic monomers, e.g., diatrizoate, iothalamate, metrizoate.
- Nonionic monomers, e.g., iohexol, iopamidol, iomeron.
- Ionic dimer, e.g., ioxaglate.
- Nonionic dimer, e.g., iodixanol, iotrolan.

Nonionic monomer contrast (iohexol, iopamidol or iomeron) is a water-soluble radiographic contrast media. It is provided as a sterile, pyrogen-free and colorless to pale-yellow solution sensitive to light and therefore should be protected from exposure. Its injection is hypertonic as compared to plasma and cerebrospinal fluid.

Organic iodine compounds block X-rays as they pass through the body, thereby allowing body structures containing iodine to be delineated in contrast to those structures that do not contain iodine. The degree of opacity produced by these compounds is directly proportional to the total amount (concentration and volume) of the iodinated contrast agent in the path of the X-rays. After intrathecal administration into the subarachnoid space, diffusion of iohexol in the CSF allows the visualization of the subarachnoid spaces of the head and spinal canal. After intravascular administration, nonionic contrast makes those vessels in its path of flow opaque, allowing visualization of the internal structures until significant hemodilution occurs.

Uses: It is used intrathecally for myelography and in contrast enhancement for computerized tomography of head and body imaging. It is used for angiocardiography, aortography including aortic root, aortic arch, ascending aorta, abdominal aorta and branches; IV digital subtraction angiography of head, neck, abdominal, renal and peripheral vessels, peripheral arteriography and excretory urography, oral/body cavity gastrointestinal (GI) tract, arthrography, hysterosalpingography (HSG).

It is excreted mainly by renal system. In patients with impaired renal function, the elimination is prolonged depending upon the degree of impairment, thus, resulting in prolonged plasma levels of contrast.

Patients sensitive to iodine may be sensitive to nonionic monomer contrast also. Adverse effects may vary directly with the concentration of the agent, the amount and technique used, and the underlying pathology. Increase in osmolality, volume, concentration, viscosity, and rate of administration of the solution may increase the incidence and severity of adverse effects. Most of the adverse effects are usually self-limited and of short duration. Overall incidence of adverse effects with nonionic contrast agents are less than with ionic contrast agents.

The amount of contrast required is usually 1–2 mL/kg body weight. Normal osmolality of human serum is 290 mOsm/kg. Ionic contrast media have much higher osmolality than normal human serum and are known as high osmolar contrast media (HOCM), while nonionic contrast media have lower osmolality than normal human serum and are known as low osmolar contrast media (LOCM).

Following intravascular iodinated agent arterial opacification takes place at approximately 20 seconds with venous peak at approximately 70 seconds. The level then declines and the contrast is finally excreted by the kidneys. These different phases of enhancement are used to image various organs depending on the indication. Spiral CT, being faster is able to acquire images during each phase, thus provide much more information.

ORAL CONTRAST

The bowel is usually opacified in CT examinations of the abdomen and pelvis as the attenuation value of the bowel is similar to the surrounding structures and as a result pathological lesions can be obscured. Materials used include are barium or iodine based preparations, which are given to the patient to drink preceding the examination to opacify the gastrointestinal tract.

Iodine containing oral contrast agents like Gastrografin and Trazograf are given for evaluating gastrointestinal tract on CT scan.

Air

Air is used as a negative per rectal contrast medium in large bowel during CT abdomen and during CT colonography.

Carbon Dioxide

Rarely carbon dioxide is used for infradiaphragmatic CT angiography in patients who are sensitive to iodinated contrast.

Adverse Reactions to Iodinated Contrast Media

Adverse reactions to iodinated contrast media (ICM) are classified as idiosyncratic and nonidiosyncratic.

Idiosyncratic Reactions

Idiosyncratic reactions typically begin within 20 minutes of the ICM injection, independent of the dose that is administered. A severe idiosyncratic reaction can occur after an injection of less than 1 mL of a contrast agent. Idiosyncratic reactions to ICM are called anaphylactic reactions.

Mild symptoms include the following: Scattered urticaria, which is the most commonly reported adverse reaction; pruritus; rhinorrhea; nausea, brief retching, and/or vomiting; diaphoresis; coughing; and dizziness. Patients with mild symptoms should be observed for examination of the lower gastrointestinal tract. They provide better delineation of mucosal details and are less expensive than water-soluble iodinated contrast media. The elimination rate is a function of gastrointestinal transit time. After GI application, it leaves the body with the feces. For CT scan of abdomen, 1000 to 1500 mL of 1 to 5% w/vol barium sulphate suspension can be used.

When intestinal perforation is suspected, a water-soluble iodinated contrast medium such as gastrografin may be used; when there is a possibility of aspiration, a nonionic water-soluble contrast medium is preferable.

Contraindications of barium sulfate products in case of known or suspected:
- Obstruction of the colon
- Gastrointestinal tract perforation
- Obstructing lesions of the small intestine
- Inflammation or neoplastic lesions of the rectum
- Hypersensitivity to barium sulfate formulations
- Recent rectal biopsy
- Pyloric stenosis.

Adverse reactions are rare. Rarely mediastinal leakage can lead to fibrosing mediastinitis while peritoneal leakage can cause adhesive peritonitis.

Nonidiosyncratic Reactions

Nonidiosyncratic reactions include the following: Bradycardia, hypotension, and vasovagal reactions; neuropathy; cardiovascular reactions; extravasation; and delayed reactions. Other nonidiosyncratic reactions include sensations of warmth, a metallic taste in the mouth, and nausea and vomiting.

- **Bradycardia, hypotension, and vasovagal reactions:** By inducing systemic parasympathetic activity, ICM can precipitate bradycardia and peripheral vasodilatation. The end result is systemic hypotension with bradycardia. This may be accompanied by other autonomic manifestations including nausea, vomiting, diaphoresis, sphincter dysfunction, and mental status changes. Untreated, these effects can lead to cardiovascular collapse and death. Some vasovagal reactions may be a result of coexisting circumstances such as emotion, apprehension, pain, and abdominal compression, rather than ICM administration.
- **Nephropathy:** Contrast agent-related nephropathy is an elevation of the serum creatinine level that is more than 0.5 mg% or more than 50% of the baseline level at 1 to 3 days after the ICM injection. The elevation peaks by 3 to 7 days, and the creatinine level usually returns to baseline in 10 to 14 days. The incidence of contrast agent-related nephropathy in the general population is estimated to be 2 to 7%. As many as 25% of patients with this

nephropathy have a sustained reduction in renal function, most commonly when the nephropathy is oliguric.

The mechanism of this type of nephropathy is thought to be a combination of pre-existing hemodynamic alterations; renal vasoconstriction, possibly through mediators such endothelin and adenosine; and direct ICM cellular toxicity. Patients with preexisting renal insufficiency have 5 to 10 times the risk of ICM-related nephropathy. Patients whose renal failure is the result of diabetic nephropathy are at the greatest risk. Azotemic diabetic patients also have the highest incidence of irreversible renal deterioration. In general, the higher the pre-existing serum creatinine level, the greater the likelihood of contrast agent–induced nephrotoxicity.

- **Cardiovascular reactions:** ICM can cause hypotension and bradycardia. Vasovagal reactions, a direct negative inotropic effect on the myocardium, and peripheral vasodilatation probably contribute to these effects. The latter 2 effects may represent the actions of cardioactive and vasoactive substances that are released after the anaphylactic reaction to the ICM. This effect is generally self-limiting, but it can also be an indicator of a more severe, evolving reaction.
- **Extravasation:** Extravasation of ICM into soft tissues during an injection can lead to tissue damage as a result of direct toxicity of the contrast agent or pressure effects, such as compartment syndrome.
- **Delayed reactions:** Delayed reactions become apparent at least 30 minutes after but within 7 days of the ICM injection. These reactions are identified in as many as 14 to 30% of patients after the injection of ionic monomers and in 8 to 10% of patients after the injection of nonionic monomers.

Common delayed reactions include the development of flu-like symptoms, such as the following: Fatigue, weakness, upper respiratory tract congestion, fevers, chills, nausea, vomiting, diarrhea, abdominal pain, pain in the injected extremity, rash, dizziness, and headache.

Treatment of Adverse Reactions

Most acute severe adverse reactions to ICM occur within 20 minutes of injection. For this reason, the patient should be monitored for a minimum of 20 minutes after an ICM injection.

Rooms in which contrast material is administered should be stocked with appropriate basic and advanced life support monitoring equipment and drugs. The equipment should be regularly checked.

Principles of treatment of adverse reaction involves mainly five basic steps: **ABCDE**

A – Maintain proper airway.
B – Breathing—support for adequate breathing.
C – Maintain adequate circulation. Obtain an IV access.
D – Use of appropriate drugs like antihistaminics for urticaria, atropine for vasovagal hypotension and bradycardia, beta-agonists for bronchospasm, hydrocortisone, etc.
E – Always have emergency back-up ready including ICU care.

Treatment of Anaphylactic Reactions

A respiratory component to an adverse reaction requires more aggressive therapy. Oxygen administration 10 to 12 L/min should be considered in any patient with respiratory difficulty. If bronchospasm is accelerating or severe, if it does not respond to inhalers, or if an upper airway edema (including laryngospasm) is present, epinephrine should be injected promptly. Intravenous use of epinephrine is optional in normotensive patients, but it is necessary in hypotensive patients with respiratory reactions.

H_1 antihistamines, such as diphenhydramine, and H_2-receptor blockers, such as cimetidine, do not have a major role in the treatment of respiratory reactions, but they may be administered after epinephrine.

Hypotension resulting from an anaphylactic reaction is treated with an intravenous iso-osmolar fluid (i.e., normal saline, Ringer lactate solution) in large volumes. Several liters of fluid may be required. If fluid and oxygen are unsuccessful in reversing the patient's hypotension, the use of vasopressors should be considered. The most specifically effective vasopressor is dopamine; at infusion rates of 2 to 10 µg/kg/min, the cerebral, renal, and splanchnic vessels remain dilated, whereas the peripheral vessels constrict. Epinephrine is less useful, its results are less predictable, and it has more adverse effects.

Urticaria

In asymptomatic patients, no treatment is needed.

In patient with symptomatic urticaria that is mild or moderate, diphenhydramine 50 mg may be administered intramuscularly, or intravenously.

In severe cases, treatment is as above; consider adding cimetidine 300 mg by slow intravenous injection or ranitidine 50 mg by slow intravenous injection.

Bronchospasm

For mild bronchospasm, treatment includes oxygen 10–12 L by face mask, close observation, and/or 2 puffs of an albuterol or metaproterenol inhaler.

For moderate cases without hypotension, treatment is as above, with epinephrine (1:1000), 0.1 to 0.3 mL given subcutaneously, repeated every 10 to 15 minutes as needed until 1 mL is administered.

In patients with severe bronchospasm, administer epinephrine (1:1000), 1 mL slow intravenous injection over approximately 5 minutes, repeated every 5 to 10 minutes as needed.

Laryngeal Edema

For mild to moderate laryngeal edema, treatment includes oxygen 10 to 12 L by face mask and epinephrine (1:1000), 0.1 to 0.3 mL given subcutaneously, repeated every 10 to 15 minutes as needed until 1 mL is administered.

In moderate to severe cases, consider calling a code or intubating the patient. Consider adding diphenhydramine 50 mg slow intravenous injection and cimetidine 300 mg slow intravenous injection or ranitidine 50 mg slow intravenous injection.

Unresponsive Patient

In unresponsive patients, defibrillation may be needed to treat ventricular fibrillation and pulseless ventricular tachycardia.
- ❖ Administer basic life support
- ❖ Treatment of nonidiosyncratic reactions.

Extravasation Injuries

Extravasation injuries are treated by elevating the affected extremity and applying cold compression. A plastic surgeon should be consulted if the patient's pain gradually increases over 2 to 4 hours, if skin blistering or ulceration develops, or if the circulation or sensation changes at or distal to the level of the extravasation. No specific treatment is unequivocally effective; therefore, most extravasation injuries are conservatively treated with supportive measures.

CHAPTER 27

CT Myelography

CT myelography provides excellent spatial resolution, detailed anatomic depiction of bone, subarachnoid space with the cord and functional imaging of the subarachnoid space. It remains an important diagnostic modality in evaluation of the spine and plays a crucial role in demonstrating spinal disease when MRI is contraindicated or inadequate or high-resolution functional spine imaging is required.

It combines the advantages of myelography and the high resolution of CT. It provides a detailed delineation of pathologic spine conditions, especially those involving the thecal sac and its contents. However, the role of CT myelography has dramatically and appropriately decreased with the advent of MRI, which provides a noninvasive method to demonstrate pathologic spine conditions with high signal intensity in soft tissues.

A spinal needle is introduced into the spinal canal to inject contrast under X-ray guidance. This is followed by a CT scan. Complications are headache, allergic reactions to contrast, nerve injury, leakage of spinal fluid and seizure. After the procedure, head is kept slightly elevated for 6 hours with 1–2 pillows on the bed.

CT myelography is used mainly to assess for spinal cord lesions and spinal canal stenosis when MRI is contraindicated or when dynamic imaging is required. Also for dorsal thoracic arachnoid web, intrathecal cysts, spinal CSF leaks, arachnoiditis or after surgery with hardware, as this hardware can cause a lot of artifact on MRI.

CHAPTER 28

CT Angiography

CT angiography (CTA) sequence is created subsequent to intravenous contrast. Images are acquired in the arterial phase and then reconstructed and exhibited in 2D or 3D format. This performance is used for imaging the aorta, renal, cerebral, coronary and peripheral arteries **(Figs. 1 to 3)**.

CT is readily available in most hospitals and stand-alone CT centers. It is fast imaging modality and provides with cross-sectional high-resolution images. Data acquired on axial scans can be used for multiplanar and 3D reconstructions. It detects subtle differences between body tissues. However, it uses X-rays which have radiation hazards, CT needs contrast media for enhanced soft tissue contrast. Contrast is contraindicated in asthma, cardiac disease, renal and certain thyroid conditions.

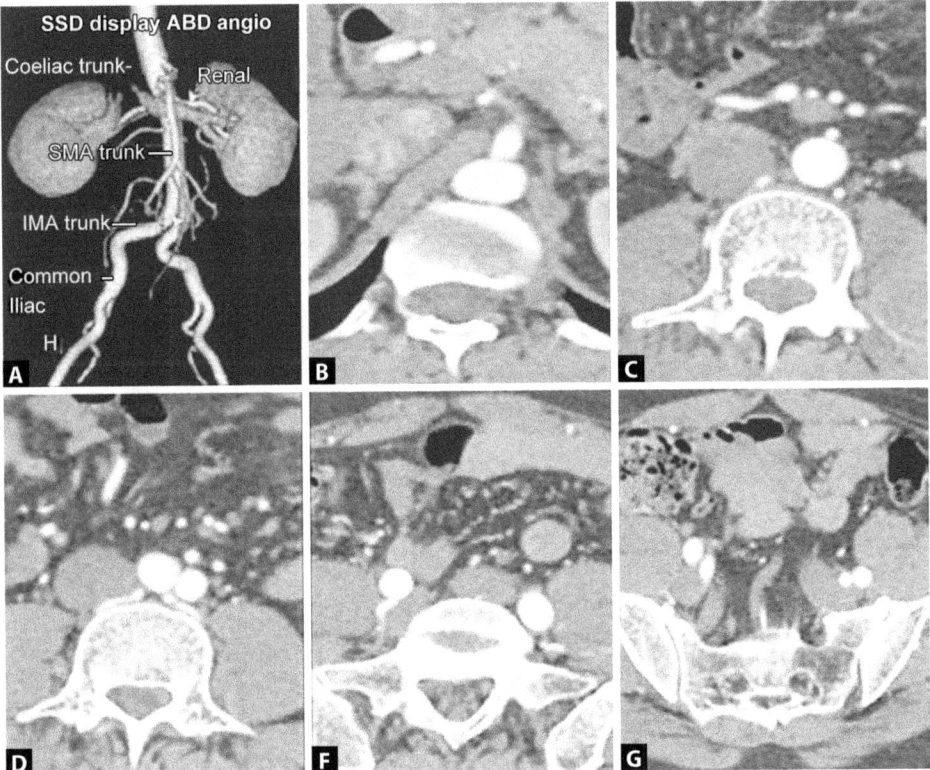

Figs. 1A to F: CT abdominal angiography.

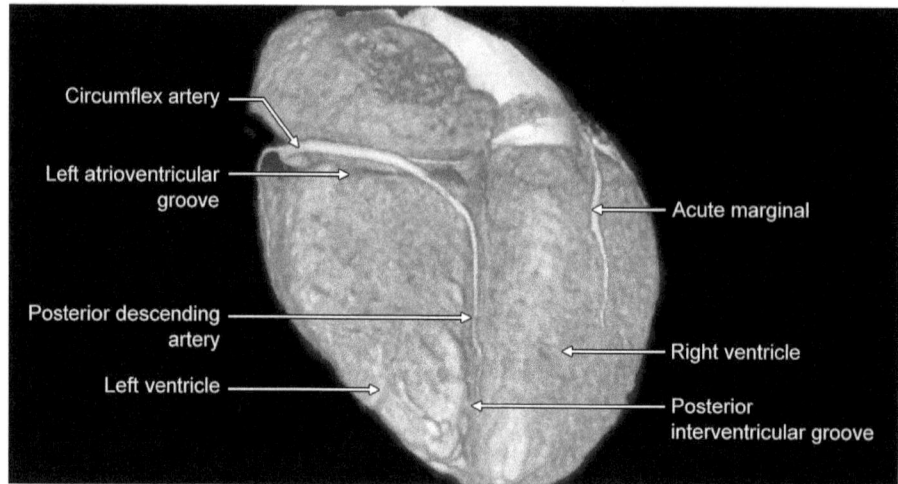

Fig. 2: Volume rendered image posterior coronal plane shows coronary arteries.

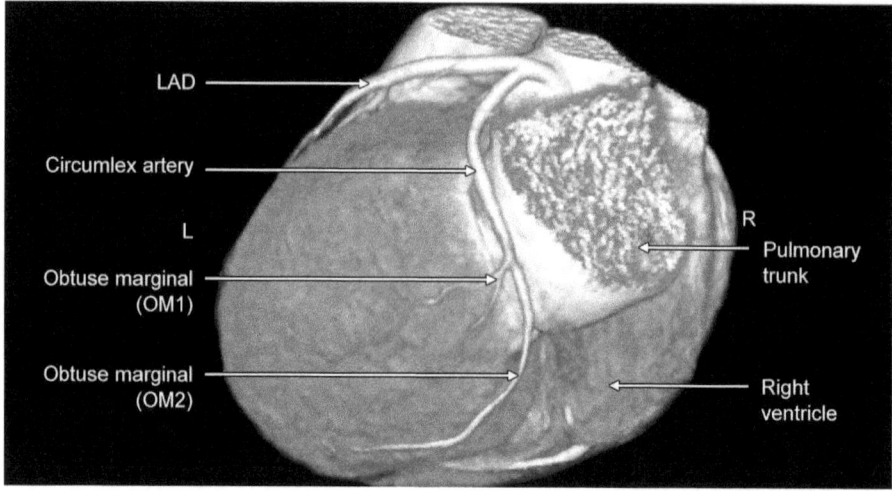

Fig. 3: Volume rendered image posterior oblique coronal plane shows coronary arteries.

Artifacts

CHAPTER 29

An artifact is an abnormal appearing false finding in an image and is unrelated to the patient. It is thus a ghost appearance and in reality it does not exist.

Motion artifacts occur due to patient's motion, implants or ornaments give rise to streak artifacts or beam hardening artifacts due to which adjacent structural details are obscured. Ring artifacts occur due to problems in detectors. When a partial volume is sampled or included in the field of view of imaging it gives rise to partial volume artifact.

- Angulation artifact is seen as the asymmetric appearance of frontal horns of lateral ventricles as head was not symmetrically positioned. In reality, both ventricles are equal in size and are symmetrical **(Fig. 1A)**.
- Ring artifacts occur as a result of detector malfunction which could either be due to improper calibration or due to detector-data ring mismatch. The center of the detector arc is the most sensitive region where ring artifacts can occur **(Fig. 1B)**.
- Motion artifact due to accidental motion of right hand by patient **(Fig. 1C)**.
- Streak artifacts due to metallic implant in tibia **(Fig. 1D)**.

Extrinsic artifacts in the form of **clothing, jewelry** or **splints** are an occasional feature on CT imaging examinations, infrequently it has been found that women keeping their brassieres on, being recognized by metallic clips **(Figs. 2A and B)**. Extrinsic artifacts are recognized for what they are by the reporting radiologist.

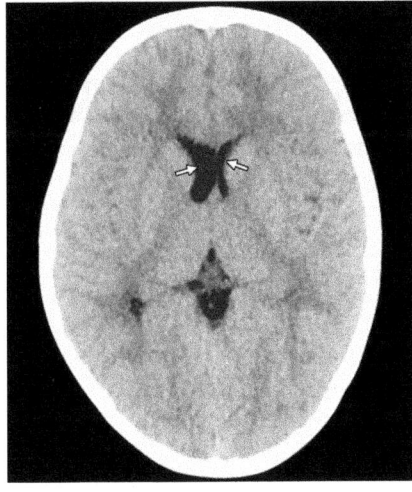

Fig. 1A: Angulation artifact.

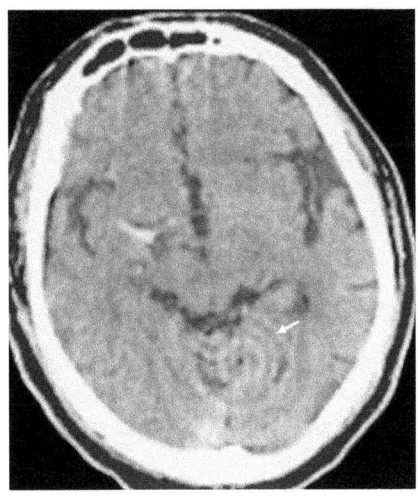

Fig. 1B: Ring artifact.

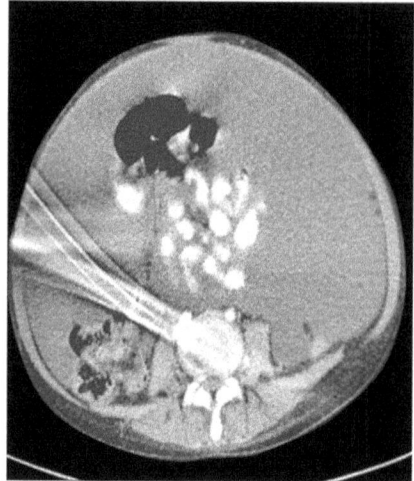

Fig. 1C: Motion artifact.

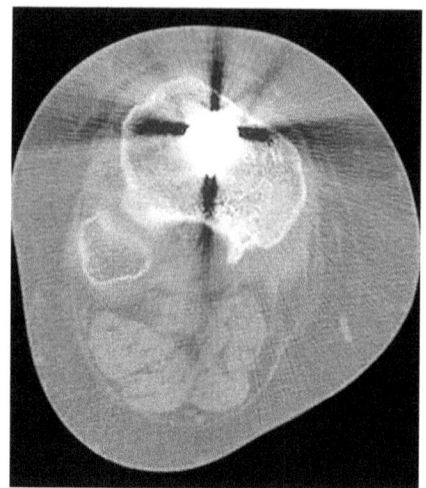

Fig. 1D: Streak artifact.

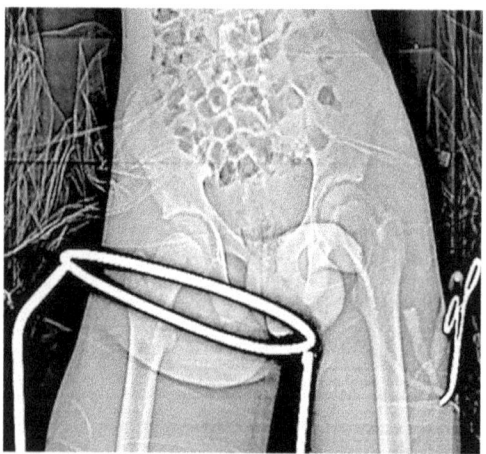

Fig. 2A: Right thigh in Thomas splint.

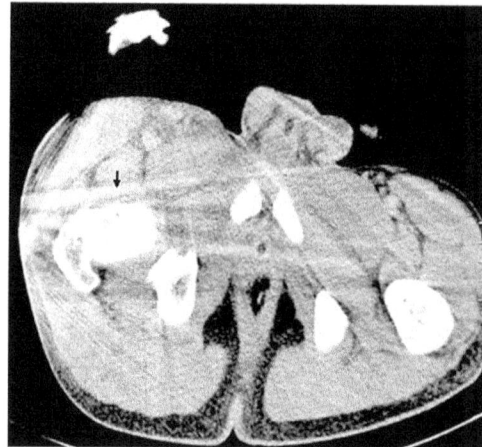

Fig. 2B: Streak artifact seen as hyperdense streaks due to reverberation from metallic Thomas splint.

PARTIAL VOLUME ARTIFACT

Partial volume artifacts seen when tissues with different absorption properties occupy the same voxel, the beam is attenuated on basis of average of attenuation values of all those tissues. This volume averaging leads to partial volume artifacts. Common sites are posterior fossa and lung diaphragm interface.

Symmetric hyperdensities seen in the frontal region are due to partial volume of the bone (**Figs. 3A and B**).

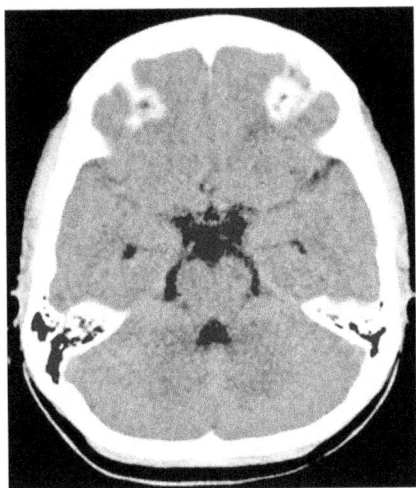

Fig. 3A: Hyperdensities seen in the frontal region are due to partial volume of the bone.

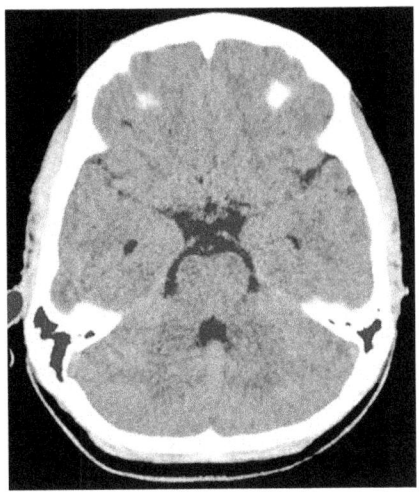

Fig. 3B: Partial volume artifact seen in frontal region.

Chapter 30

Thermoluminescent Dosimeter

Thermoluminescent dosimeter (TLD) measures ionizing radiation exposure by measuring the amount of visible light emitted from crystal in the detector when the crystal is heated **(Fig. 1)**. The amount of light emitted is dependent upon the radiation exposure.

Materials exhibiting thermoluminescence in response to ionizing radiation include calcium fluoride, calcium sulfate, calcium borate, lithium fluoride, lithium borate, potassium bromide, and feldspar. When a TLD is exposed to ionizing radiation at ambient temperatures, the radiation interacts with the phosphor crystal and deposits all or part of the incident energy in that material. Some of the atoms in the material that absorb that energy become ionized, producing free electrons and areas lacking one or more electrons called holes. Imperfections in the crystal lattice structure act as sites where free electrons can become trapped and locked into place.

Heating the crystal causes the crystal lattice to vibrate, releasing the trapped electrons in the process. Released electrons return to the original ground state, releasing the captured energy from ionization as light, hence the name thermoluminescent. Released light is counted using photomultiplier tubes and the number of photons counted is proportional to the quantity of radiation striking the phosphor.

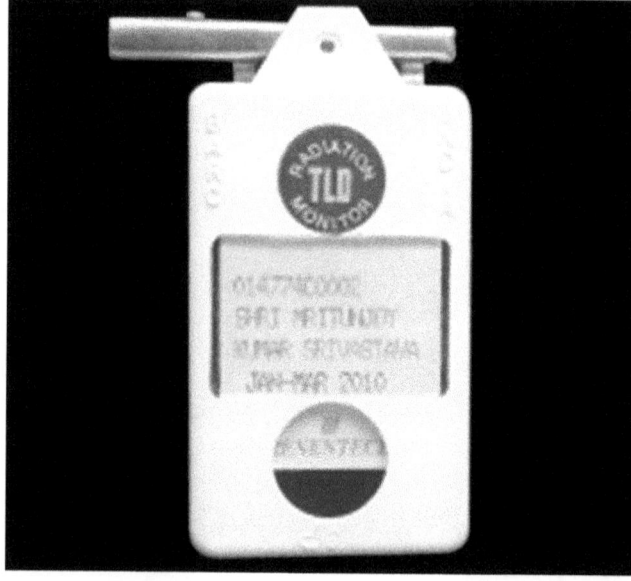

Fig. 1: Thermoluminescent dosimeter.

Thermoluminescent dosimeter (TLD) **(Fig. 1)** is worn for a period of time (usually 3 months or less) and then must be processed to determine the dose received, if any. Thermoluminescent dosimeters can measure doses as low as 1 millirem. The advantages of a TLD over other personnel monitors are its linearity of response to dose, its relative energy independence, and its sensitivity to low doses. It is also reusable, which is an advantage over film badges. However, no permanent record or re-readability is provided and an immediate, on the job readout is not possible.

Diagnosis on CT Images (Representative Cases)

CHAPTER 31

PANCREATITIS (FIG. 1)

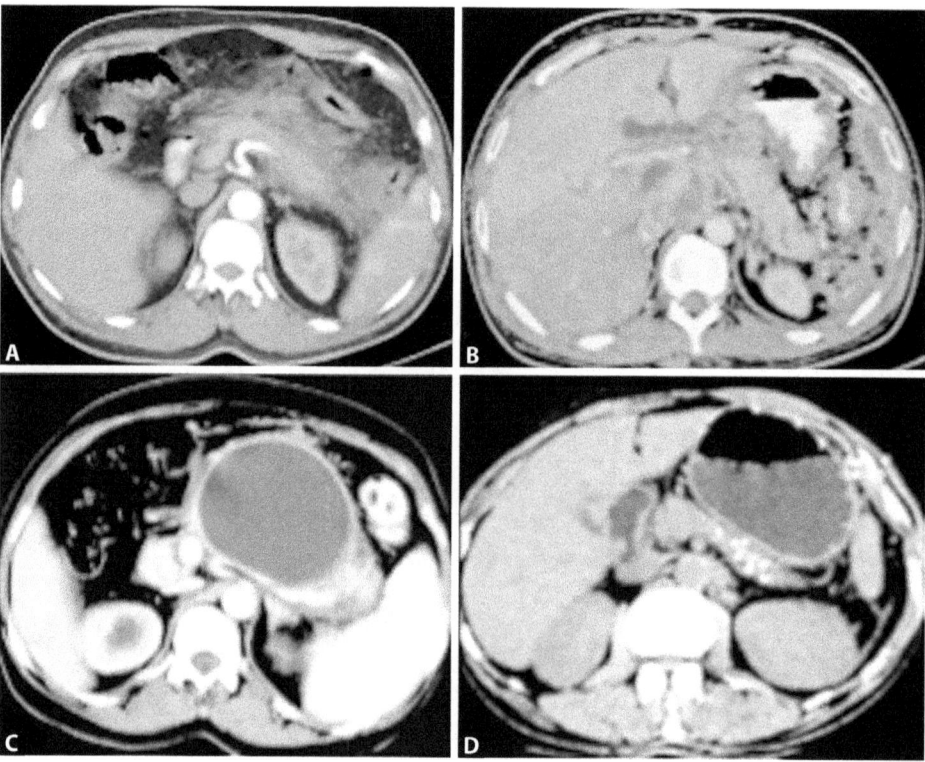

Figs. 1A to D: (A) Pancreas is bulky with extensive peripancreatic fat stranding which also extends to Gerota fascia and perirenal fat; (B) Parenchymal interstitial edema presence of parenchymal necrosis, retroperitoneal fat necrosis; (C) Contrast CT abdomen shows a hypodense pseudocyst of pancreas with thick enhancing walls in the lesser sac anterior to the body and tail of pancreas which are barely perceptible; (D) Axial CT abdomen shows chronic atrophic pancreatitis with speckled to nodular calcification in the tail and body of pancreas.

URINARY BLADDER DIVERTICULUM WITH LARGE CALCULUS AND STAGHORN CALCULI RIGHT KIDNEY (FIG. 2)

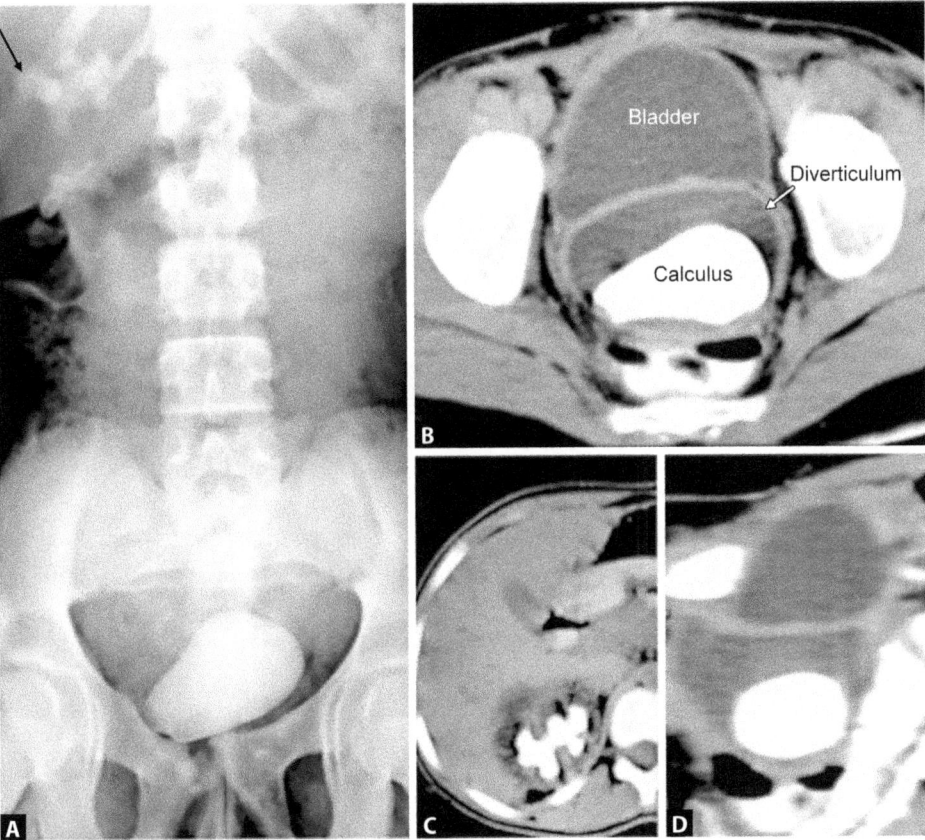

Figs. 2A to D: (A) Plain X-ray abdomen shows multiple staghorn calculi in right kidney and a large calculus in bladder area; (B) CT scan demonstrates a large posterior bladder diverticulum with a large calculus; (C) The large staghorn calculus in right kidney; (D) Sagittal recon CT image shows a posterior diverticulum filled with urine and a large calculus within it.

BICONVEX EXTRADURAL HEMATOMA (TWO DIFFERENT CASES) (FIG. 3)

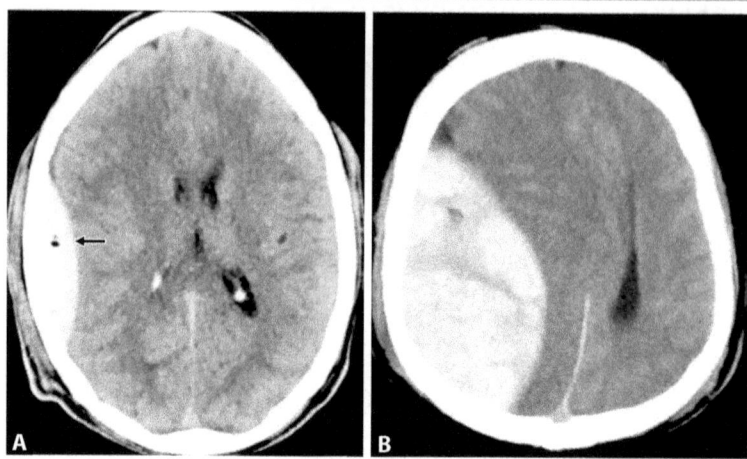

Figs. 3A and B: (A) Plain CT brain shows right biconvex extradural hematoma with small loculated air inside (arrow); (B) In another case CT brain shows a massive right biconvex extradural hematoma with significant mass effect on adjacent brain parenchyma and ventricular system.

TORTUOUS THORACIC AORTA (FIG. 4)

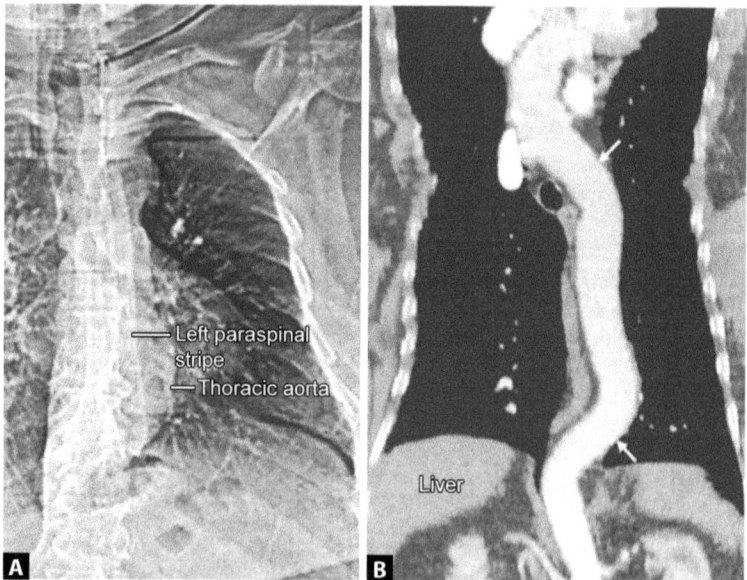

Figs. 4A and B: (A) Topo CT image of chest shows prominent descending aorta raising a suspicion of aneurysm; (B) Aortic reconstruction following contrast CT of chest and abdomen shows no aneurysm but only tortuous and elongated dilatation of thoracic aorta (arrows).

LARGE DESCENDING THORACIC AORTA ANEURYSM (FIG. 5)

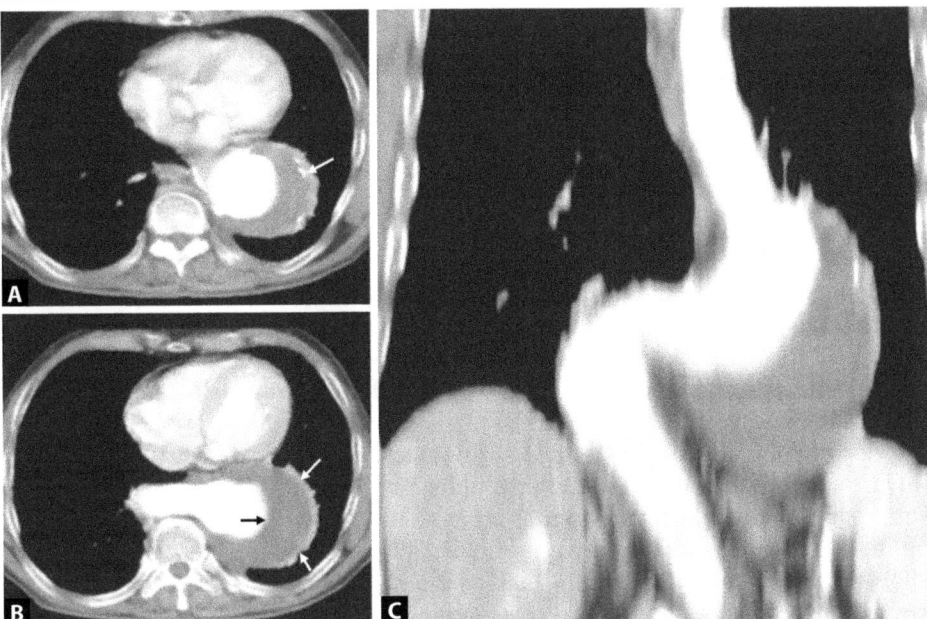

Figs. 5A to C: Contrast enhanced CT scan (A and B) axial sections; (C) Coronal reformatted image shows a large descending thoracic aorta aneurysm with a large component of intramural thrombus (arrows) which shows no contrast uptake. Calcification is present in the wall abutting the thrombus.

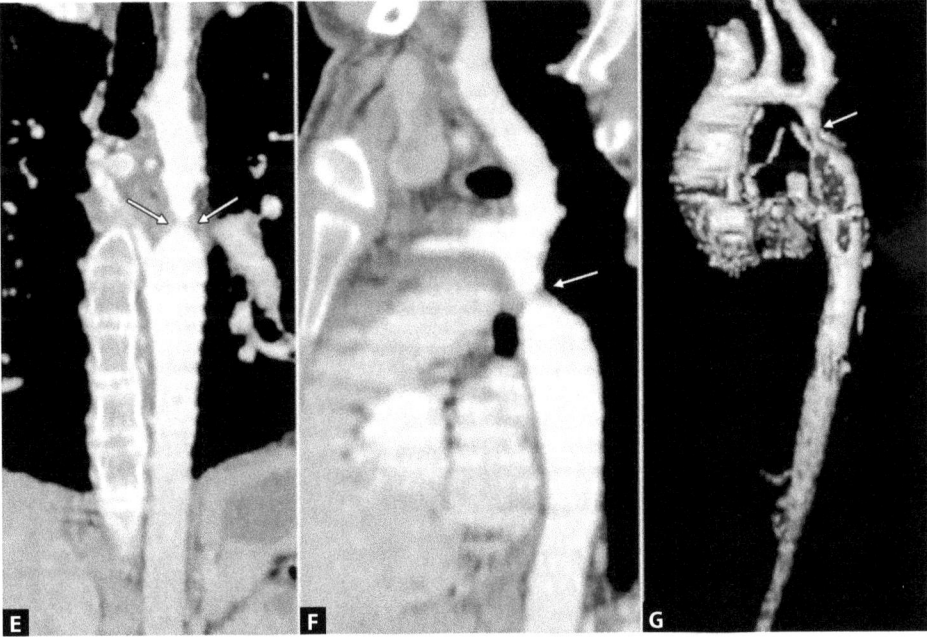

Figs. 5E to G: (E and F) Coronal and sagittal reformatted image shows the actual site of coarctation (arrows); (G) CT angiogram shows exact location of narrowing (arrow).

Interventional Radiology

CHAPTER 32

Interventional radiology is fast growing branch of medicine. Interventional procedures are first step towards pinhole surgery. The guide wires and catheters **(Figs. 1 and 2)** are put under the guidance of digital subtraction angiography (DSA), computed tomography (CT), ultrasonography or X-ray in the desired place in the body and further work is done. Most of the procedures are done under local anesthesia.

The principle of interventional radiology (IR) is to diagnose or treat the disease using the least invasive technique. In IR, fluoroscopy, ultrasound, CT, and MRI are used to advance a catheter or probe into the body to diagnose or treat the disease. Images direct interventional procedures, which are usually done with needles and catheters. The images provide pathway that allow guiding the tools through the body to the area of pathology. This minimize trauma, reduce infection and grossly reduces recovery time.

Common IR procedures are:
* Biopsy of a tissue sample from the area of interest is taken for pathological examination from a percutaneous approach.

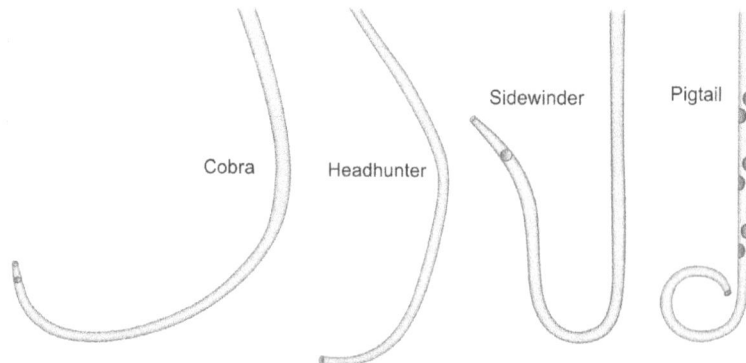

Fig. 1: Angiographic catheters in multiple preformed shapes—Cobra; Headhunter; Sidewinder; Pigtail for selective angiography.

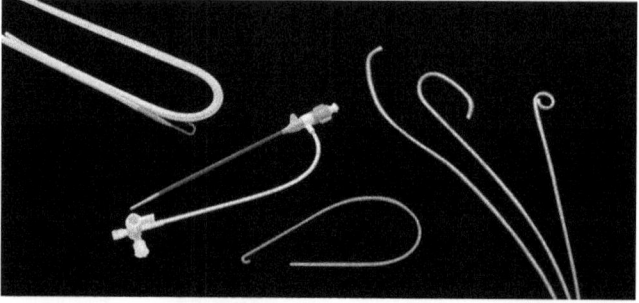

Fig. 2: Catheters and sheaths.

Chapter 32: Interventional Radiology

- In nephrostomy placement of a catheter directly into the kidney to drain urine in situations where normal flow of urine is obstructed. Through nephrostomy, nephroureteral stents can be placed through the ureter and into the bladder.
- In biliary intervention catheters are placed in the biliary system to bypass biliary obstructions for decompression of biliary system. Permanent biliary stents are also positioned.
- In cholecystostomy tube is placed into the gallbladder to remove infected bile in patients with cholecystitis, who are too weak or too sick to undergo surgery.
- In angiography the blood vessels are mapped to look for abnormalities with the use of iodinated contrast and gadolinium-based agents.
- In balloon angioplasty the narrow or blocked blood vessels are dilated using a balloon; followed by placement of self-expanding metallic stents.
- In embolization abnormal blood vessels are blocked to stop bleeding. A variety of embolic agents are used, including alcohol, glue, metallic coils, polyviny alcohol particles.
- In thrombolysis the blood clots are dissolved with both pharmaceutical and mechanical means.
- In chemoembolization—cancer treatment is straight delivered to a tumor through its blood supply.
- In radioembolization, the radioactive microspheres are delivered to the tumor to kill the tumor cells while minimizing exposure to healthy cells.

A variety of catheters are used in interventional radiology that include catheters, microcatheters, drainage catheters, balloon catheters and central venous catheters.

IR procedures are performed on an outpatient basis or may require a short hospital stay. General anesthesia generally is not required. Complications, pain and recovery time are substantially reduced and the procedures are less expensive than surgery.

Anterior mediastinal tumors like thymic cyst **(Figs. 3 and 4)**, thymic, lymphatic, or germ cell tumors are easily accessible to needle biopsy.

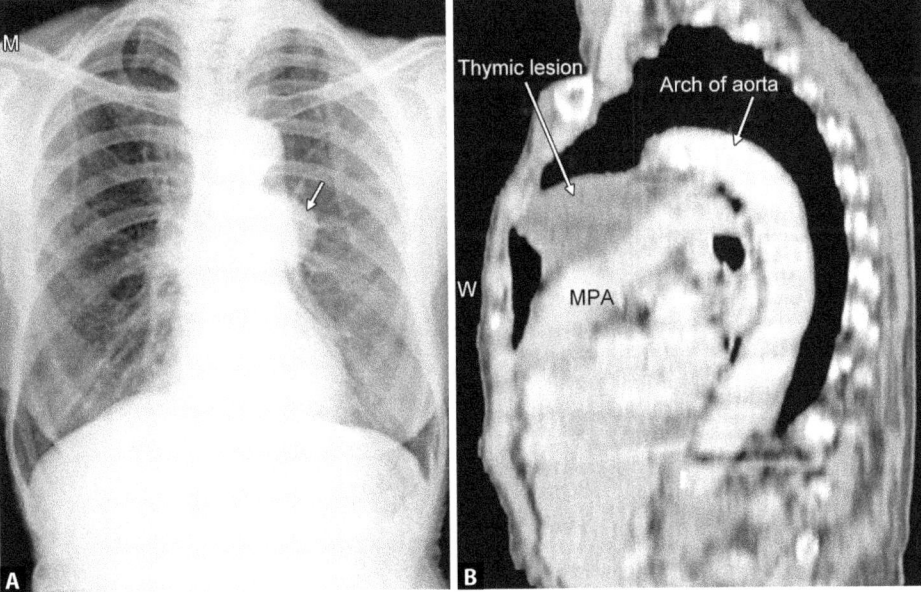

Figs. 3A and B: (A) Chest X-ray of a 56-year-old female shows anterior mediastinal left parahilar rounded opacity; (B) CT chest coronal reconstruction revealed a 4.4 X 5.8 cm well-defined unilocular cystic lesion (CT value 16 HU) in anterior mediastinum in the region of thymus on left side. The lesion had thin enhancing wall suggestive of thymic cyst. No evidence of calcification, mediastinal or hilar adenopathy was seen.

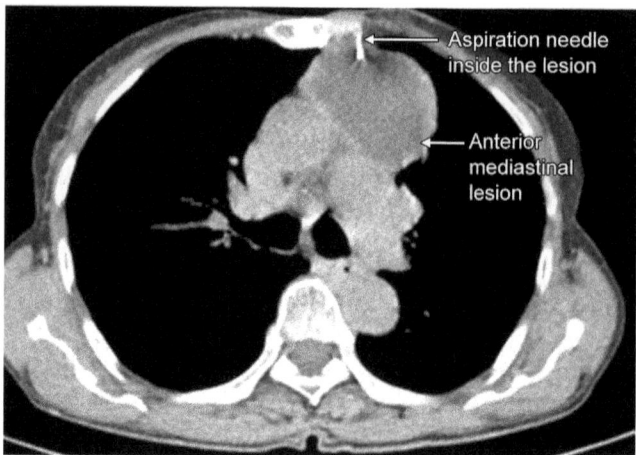

Fig. 4: Same case as **Figure 3,** CT guided aspiration was done and 5 cc of brownish fluid (suggesting some hemorrhage) was aspirated and a diagnosis of thymic cyst was confirmed.

CT GUIDED PRECISION BIOPSY

CT guided precision robotic assistance biopsy with automated planner **(Figs. 5 and 6)** reduce the number of needle passes, time spent and number of check scans which leads to significant reduction to patient's radiation dosage treated by this technique. Caroticocavernous and even vertebral AV fistula have also been treated with an ingenious detachable balloon introduced by percutaneous catheter. Dural AV fistula has also been successfully treated by embolization as have aneurysms.

Percutaneous biliary duct drainage: Patients with obstructive jaundice can be investigated by fine needle percutaneous cholangiography. Once the dilated ducts have been demonstrated, these can also be catheterized percutaneously and a drain is left *in situ* to decompress the biliary system and relieve the patient's acute symptoms.

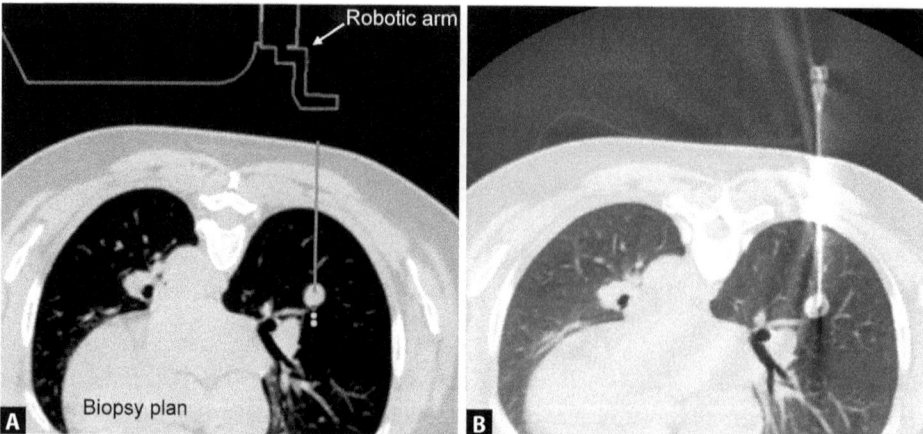

Figs. 5A and B: (A) Plan for posterior straight approach biopsy (red line) for a 12 mm nodule in right lung; (B) Check scan shows precise positioning of needle in the nodule.

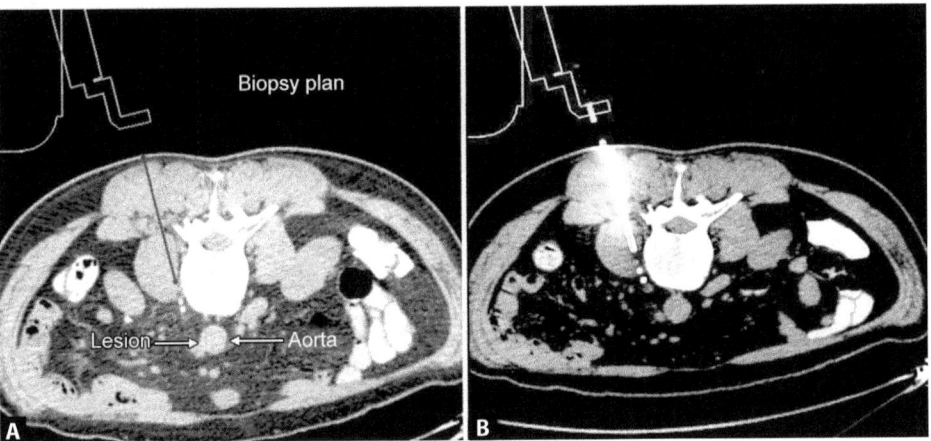

Figs. 6A and B: (A) Posterior approach biopsy plan for a 9 mm left para-aortic lymph node; (B) The needle held in robotic arm is in the process of moving into the left para-aortic lymph node.

Percutaneous removal of biliary duct stones: A major problem in the biliary tract is the patient with stones in the ducts which have not been found at operation and are later demonstrated by postoperative T-tube cholangiography.

It is possible for the radiologist to remove such stones and save the patient from a further laparotomy. A guide wire is inserted into the ducts through the T-tube tract and a catheter with a wire snare is passed over the guide wire and into the ducts. The stones can then be snared and removed through the T-tube tract.

Tips: Transjugular intrahepatic portosystemic stent (TIPS) shunting is being increasingly used to create a portosystemic shunt between hepatic and portal vein branches in the treatment and control of complications in patients with portal hypertension. The interventional radiologist uses a percutaneous transjugular approach to the liver for a procedure which previously required major surgery.

CHAPTER 33

Tidbits on CT Scan

Code blue: Code blue is defined as, any patient with an unexpected cardiac or respiratory arrest requiring resuscitation within the hospital. Activation of a hospital-wide alert is declared by telephone to administrative system by the staff where emergency has taken place.

Immediate administrative action is done, as code blue hospital announcement, that patient is having a medical emergency, usually cardiac or respiratory arrest. The announcement also tells you where the emergency is. Hospital personnel are trained to respond to code blue within 2-4 minutes. They reach the location along with emergency treatment box.

The highest slice ct scanner: The highest slice CT scanner is the Aquilion One with 640-slices. It has the newest technology that enables faster and more detailed diagnosis.

Deep learning reconstruction: Deep Learning Reconstruction (DLR) is the future of CT providing the elusive triad of low-dose, high-quality, and high-speed, which can be tailored to the needs of individual patients whilst producing a natural-appearing image. DLR has redefined the definition of ultra-low-dose CT into the realms of plain radiography.

Dark field computed tomography: Dark field CT (DFCT) is an advanced medical imaging technique that has gained prominence recently for its ability to provide high-contrast and detailed images of biological tissues.

Triple-phase CT: The triple-phase liver CT protocol is a useful examination in the assessment of focal liver lesions, hypervascular liver metastases and endocrine tumors. It involves a dedicated late arterial phase, portal venous phase and delayed phase acquisition.

Pitch in CT scan: The pitch in multislice spiral CT is defined as the ratio of the table increment over the detector collimation in this study. In parallel to the current framework for studying longitudinal image resolution, the central fan-beam rays of direct and opposite directions are considered, assuming a narrow cone-beam angle.

Sixth generation CT: It helical and spiral CT, in this technique the data are continuously acquired or collected without pausing while the patient is simultaneously transported at a constant speed through the gantry.

Difference between slice thickness and interval in CT: In helical CT, slice thickness and reconstruction interval are independent. Slice thickness is determined by the detector width and pitch, while reconstruction interval can be chosen arbitrarily. The narrower the reconstruction interval, the better is 3D reconstructions.

Gantry tilt: The gantry tilt is the angle between the vertical plane, and the plane containing the X-ray beam and the detector array. The gantry angulation allows aligning the selected anatomic region with the scanning plane. A CT gantry can typically be angled up to 30° forward or backward.

Newest CT scanner: The new NAEOTOM Alpha is distinct from conventional computed tomography (CT) scanners. It utilizes cutting-edge photon-counting technology to deliver drastic improvements in image resolution and contrast, which can lead to earlier detection and greater clarity in diagnosis.

WINDOWS: The meaning or full form of WINDOWS is Wide Interactive Network Development for Office Work Solution.

CHAPTER 34

CT Scan versus MRI Scan

CT scan uses ionizing radiation like X-rays whereas MRI scans use a strong magnetic field and radiofrequency energy. The difference between CT and MRI scans are mentioned in **Table 1**.

Table 1: The difference between CT scan and MRI scan.

CT scan	MRI
CT scans take a fast series of X-ray pictures, which are put together to create images of the area scanned.	MRI uses strong magnetic fields to take pictures of the inside of the body.
CT scans are usually the first choice for imaging.	MRI is useful for certain diseases that a CT scan cannot detect.
A CT scan is better for: • Showing bone and joint issues. • Blood clots. • Some organ injuries.	MRI is better for: • Tumors. • Ligaments and soft tissue injuries. • Joint injury or diseases. • Spinal injury or diseases. • Injury or disease of internal organs.
CT scan provides better spatial resolution. That means CT scans are good at showing the edges, where one structure ends and the other one begins.	MRI provides better contrast resolution.
CT scans are performed to help diagnose tumors, investigate internal bleeding, or check for other internal injuries or damage. CT can also be used for a tissue biopsy or fluid aspiration.	MRI scan provides clear and detailed images of soft tissue. Bones are not visualized very well, since bone tissue does not contain much water.
Disadvantages of CT scans include the risks from exposure to ionizing radiation and possible reactions to the contrast agent.	Disadvantages of MRI are claustrophobia because it is a small enclosed space, effects of magnetic field on metal devices implanted in the body and reactions to the contrast agent.

CHAPTER 35

Medical Records

The importance of keeping medical records plays a pivotal role in signifying the medical supervision of patients, for care quality, leading to reduced morbidity and mortality rates. The enhancement of quality can be achieved through the scrutiny of hospital records.

Medical records provide indisputable verification within a court of law. They are very crucial in safeguarding against accusations of neglect, inadequate service, unfair business practices, and medical misconduct.

Medical records serve as our strongest defense against allegations. Hence it is important to prioritize them. To overcome the storage problem, electronic medical record (EMR) is a viable option.

Keeping a hard copy of the medical records is essential from a medico-legal point of view in different situations. The situations are mainly:

- When a patient needs to be transferred to another hospital or referral
- For written consent
- Important points should be recorded like allergies, drug sensitivities
- Software crash or loss for whatever reason it be
- Medico-legal cases

USAGE OF EMR AND ITS ADVANTAGES

Electronic Medical Record (EMR) software streamlines record-keeping, overcoming paper-based limitations. Accessible to multiple users, it eliminates errors, adheres to legal standards, and allows seamless data sharing. It offers financial benefits by reducing transcription costs, focusing more on patients.

Patients can easily track the reports of the radiological investigations and other tests. It helps in accurate billing and appointment tracking. Integration with insurance providers and financial systems optimizes claim processing. EMR software efficiently manages healthcare centers, serving as a knowledgeable, all-encompassing system. It integrates departments, grants 24 × 7 access, and curbing errors effectively.

CHAPTER 36

Radiation Units

Rad (radiation absorbed dose) is a unit used to measure quantity of absorbed dose. This relates to the amount of energy actually absorbed in some material, and is used for any type of radiation and any material. One rad is defined as the absorption of 100 ergs per gram of material.

Rem (roentgen equivalent man) is a unit used to derive quantity of equivalent dose. This relates the absorbed dose in human tissue to the effective biological damage of the radiation. Equivalent dose is often expressed in terms of thousandths of a rem or mrem. To determine equivalent dose (rem), multiply radiation absorbed dose (rad) by a quality factor (Q) that is unique to the type of incident radiation.

Gray (Gy) is a unit used to measure quantity of absorbed dose. This relates to the amount of energy actually absorbed in some material, and is used for any type of radiation and any material. One gray is equal to one joule of energy deposited in one kg of a material. Absorbed dose is often expressed in terms of hundredths of a gray, or centi-grays. One gray is equivalent to 100 rads.

Sievert (Sv) is a unit used to derive quantity equivalent dose. This relates the absorbed dose in human tissue to the effective biological damage of the radiation. Equivalent dose is often expressed in terms of millionths of a sievert, or micro-sievert. To determine equivalent dose (Sv), multiply absorbed dose (Gy) by a quality factor (Q) that is unique to the type of incident radiation. One sievert is equivalent to 100 rem.

A given material has an ability to absorb radiation when exposed. This differs with certain materials; some will absorb more, e.g., lead or less, e.g., water, as radiation passes through.

A dose of 1 rad means the absorption of 100 ergs of radiation energy per gram of absorbing material.

SI units (Système international d'unités): A dose of 1 gray means the absorption of 1 joule of radiation energy per kilogram of absorbing material.

$$1 \text{ Gy} = 100 \text{ rads}$$

The dose equivalent is a measure of biological effect for whole body irradiation. It is measured in Sievert (Sv). The dose equivalent is equal to the product of the absorbed dose and the quality factor (Q).

The quality factor depends on the type of radiation. X-ray and gamma ray the quality factor (Q) is 1.

$$1 \text{ Sievert (Sv)} = 100 \text{ rads. } 1 \text{ mSv} = 0.1 \text{ rad}$$

Radiation levels are measured mSv and other international variants as follows:
- 1 Sv = 1000 mSv = 1,000,000 µSv (microsieverts) = 100 rem = 100,000 mrem (millirem)
- 1 mSv = 100 mrem = 0.1 rem
- 1 µSv = 0.1 mrem
- 1 rem = 0.01 Sv = 10 mSv
- 1 mrem = 0.00001 Sv = 0.01 mSv = 10 µSv

1 Rad = 1 Rem, 1 rem = 0.01 Sv = 10 mSv = 10 mGy = 0.01 Gy.

CHAPTER 37

Radiation Hazards

In the environment, there is continuous radiation, which is both natural and artificial. The natural sources include cosmic radiation from space, radiation from the earth and its internal radionuclide. Artificial sources of radiation include X-ray equipment, nuclear weapons and radioactive medication.

Radiation is energy in transit in the form of high speed particles and electromagnetic waves. Radiation can be ionizing or nonionizing. X-rays are electromagnetic waves or photons not emitted from the nucleus, but normally emitted by energy changes in electrons. These energy changes are either in electron orbital shells that surround an atom or in the process of slowing down such as in an X-ray machine.

Roentgen discovered X-rays in November 1895, after that X-rays are used globally. Initial hazards of radiation reported were eye complaints and severe progressive dermatitis. Clarence E Dally developed ulcerating carcinoma of his left hand in 1896. He was involved in the production of X-ray tubes, where he was using his own hand to test their output. Delayed effects of radiation began to be documented only 20 years after their initial discovery, through individual case reports.

CLASSIFICATION OF RADIATION EFFECTS

Radiation effects are classified as: Directly proportional to dose, i.e., deterministic effects, or not directly proportional to dose, i.e., stochastic effects.

❖ Somatic
- *Deterministic effects:* Deterministic effects are related with certainty to a known dose of radiation. There is threshold to the dose of radiation. In these, the severity is dose related and include cataracts, blood dyscrasias and impaired fertility.
- *Stochastic effects:* Stochastic effects are random effects without threshold. In these, probability increases with dose, and severity may not be dose related and includes cancer and genetic effects.

Health Effects

Exposure to high levels of radiation leads to deterministic (nonstochastic) health effects. These effects depend on the dose of the radiation the person is exposed to. Greater the exposure, more severe is the damage. Short-term, high-level exposure is referred to as "acute" exposure. Health effects produced by an 'acute' exposure to radiation occur quickly. Nonstochastic health effects are mostly noncancerous. The most important health effects are burns and radiation sickness. Radiation sickness (radiation poisoning) can cause premature aging or even death. Exposure to fatal doses can lead to death.

Some symptoms of radiation sickness are nausea, weakness, hair loss, skin burns, diminished organ function.

Relatively high "bursts" of radiation that patients receive during medical treatment often cause acute effects. Neutropenia due to radiation exposure can occur.

Somatic certainty effects which have been evaluated on patients undergoing radiotherapy have shown that the tissues most sensitive to radiation damage are bone marrow, eye and gonads. From studies on radiotherapy patients, the threshold doses are estimated at 1 Gy (Gray) for bone marrow, 2–8 Gy for eye, 3–4 Gy to elicit ovulation failure in middle aged women and 6–10 Gy cause failure of spermatogenesis. It has been found that the GIT is sensitive at 75 Gy, the brain beyond 55-60 Gy, the spinal cord at 45 Gy, the heart at 40–50 Gy and the lung at 11 Gy.

Stochastic Effects

Cancer is the uncontrolled growth of cells. Cell division is a fundamental process that takes place in the human body. A multitude of mechanisms exist to ensure that this process occur error free and in strict control. Damage occurring at the cellular or molecular level can disrupt this and lead to uncontrolled proliferation of cells. Ionizing radiation has the ability to break chemical bonds in atoms and molecules. Owing to this potential, it may be referred to as a carcinogen. Cancer is commonly considered as the primary health effect from radiation exposure.

Malignancies because of radiation exposure are leukemias, carcinoma of lung, breast, thyroid and skin and meningiomas and osteosarcomas. Effects on the fetus are both deterministic and stochastic which lead to childhood malignancies. Irradiation in utero can lead to developmental abnormalities (more during 8-25 weeks of gestation), and cancer may develop during childhood or as adult.

However since radiation exposure has inherent risks of radiation effects, no decision to expose an individual can be undertaken without weighing benefits of exposure against potential risks. That is, making a benefit risk analysis.

CHAPTER 38

Radiation Protection

The International Commission of Radiation Protection (ICRP) formed in 1928. The ICRP is the international regulatory body. Atomic Energy Regulatory Board (AERB) which is the Indian regulatory board constituted on November 15, 1983. The mission of the Board is to ensure that the use of ionizing radiation and nuclear energy in India does not cause undue risk to health and environment.

AERB recommends and lays down guidelines regarding the specifications of medical X-ray equipment, for the room layout of X-ray installation, regarding the work practices in X-ray department, the protective devices and also the responsibilities of the radiation personnel, employer and Radiation Safety Officer (RSO). It is the authority in India which exercises a regulatory control and has the power to decommissioning X-ray installations and also for imposing penalties on any person contravening these rules.

THE OBJECTIVE OF RADIATION PROTECTION

Provide an appropriate standard of protection for man without unduly limiting the beneficial practices giving rise to radiation exposure. Current standards of protection are meant to prevent occurrence of deterministic effects by keeping doses below relevant thresholds and ensure that all reasonable steps are taken to reduce induction of stochastic effects.

Optimization of Protection and ALARA Principle

Optimization of protection can be achieved by optimizing the procedure to administer a radiation dose which is as low as reasonably achievable (ALARA), so as to derive maximum diagnostic information with minimum discomfort to the patient. ALARA recognizes that there will always be some radiation exposure to patients involved in radiological procedures using ionizing radiation, but it also recognizes that these exposures can be minimized.

Principles of Radiation Protection

- **Justification:** Justification of a practice, e.g., the benefit to risk ratio is high for CT brain in cerebrovascular hemorrhage and low in screening mammography in women below 35 years.
- **Optimized protection:** "Optimization of the radiological procedure" is to reduce radiation exposures to the minimum levels. This optimization is possible by good quality assurance and quality control.
- **Dose limitation:** By using high frequency generators which enable "high kV and low mAs" technique. The high kV beam has higher energy photons, which undergo a lesser degree of beam attenuation and greater penetration of the beam through the patient. Therefore the tissue deposition of photons is reduced, which reduces the radiation dose to the patient.

Triad of Radiation Protection Actions

Time

The exposure time is related to radiation exposure and exposure rate (exposure per unit time).

$$\text{Exposure} = \text{Exposure rate} \times \text{Time}$$

This implies that if the exposure time is kept short, then the resulting dose to the individual is small.

Distance

Distance is between the source of radiation and the exposed individual. The exposure to the individual decreases inversely as the square of the distance. This is known as the inverse square law. Another important consideration with respect to distance relates to the source-to-image receptor distance (SID). The appropriate SID for various examinations must always be maintained. Long SID results in less divergent beam and thus decreases the concentration of photons in the patients. Short SID results in the reverse action and increases the patient dose. Hence the longest possible SID should be employed in examinations.

Shielding

Shielding implies that certain materials (concrete, lead) will attenuate radiation when they are placed between the source of radiation and the exposed individual.

X-ray Tube Shielding (Source Shielding)

X-ray tube housing is lined with thin sheets of lead because X-rays produced in the tube are scattered in all directions. This shielding is intended to protect both patients and personnel from leakage radiation. AERB recommends a maximum allowable leakage radiation from tube housing not greater than 1 mGy per hour per 100 cm^2.

Room Shielding (Structural Shielding)

The lead lined walls of radiology department are referred to as protective barriers because they are designed to protect individuals located outside the X-ray rooms from unwanted radiation. Primary barrier is one which is directly struck by the primary or the useful beam. Secondary barrier is one which is exposed to secondary radiation either by leakage from X-ray tube or by scattered radiation from the patient.

X-ray Examination Room

The room housing an X-ray unit is not less than 18 m^2 for general purpose radiography and conventional fluoroscopy equipment. In case the installation is located in a residential complex, it is ensured that

- Wall of the X-ray rooms on which primary X-ray beam falls is not less than 35 cm thick brick or equivalent,
- Walls of the X-ray room on which scattered X-rays fall is not less than 23 cm thick brick or equivalent,
- There is a shielding equivalent to at least 23 cm thick brick or 1.7 mm lead in front of the doors and windows of the X-ray room to protect the adjacent areas, either used by general public or not under possession of the owner of the X-ray room. Unshielded openings in an

X-ray room for ventilation or natural light are located above a height of 2 m from the finished level outside the X-ray room.

Patient Waiting Area

Patient waiting areas are provided outside the X-ray room. A suitable warning signal such as red light and a warning placard is provided at a conspicuous place outside the X-ray room and kept 'ON' when the unit is in use to warn persons not connected with the particular examination from entering the room.

CT Room

The highly collimated X-ray beam in CT results in markedly non uniform distribution of absorbed dose perpendicular to the tomographic plane during the CT exposure. Therefore the size of the CT room housing the gantry of the CT unit as recommended by AERB should not be less than 25 m². The walls and viewing window of the control booth, which should have lead equivalents of 1.5 mm. The location of control booth, which should not be located where the primary beam falls directly, and the radiation should be scattered twice before entering the booth.

Personnel Shielding

Personnel should remain in the radiation environment only when necessary. The distance between the personnel and the patient should be maximized when practical as the intensity of radiation decreases as the square of distance (inverse square law).

Shielding apparel should be used as and when necessary which comprise of lead aprons, eye glasses with side shields, gloves, thyroid shields and caps which are lead lined.

Lead aprons are shielding apparel recommended for use by radiation workers. These are classified as a secondary barrier to the effects of ionizing radiation. These aprons protect an individual only from secondary (scattered) radiation, not the primary beam.

About 0.25 mm lead thickness attenuates 66% of the beam at 75 kVp and 1 mm attenuates 99% of the beam at same kVp. It is recommended that for general purpose radiography the minimum thickness of lead equivalent in the protective apparel should be 0.5 mm. When not in use, all protective apparel should be laid flat on tables and should not be hung on racks, otherwise there can be cracks or tear in protective lead sheet. Protective apparel also should be radiographed for defects such as internal cracks and tears at least once a year. It is recommended that women radiation workers should wear a customized lead apron that reaches below mid thigh level and wraps completely around the pelvis. This would eliminate an accidental exposure to a conceptus.

Lead Free Aprons (Zero Lead Aprons)

Conventional protective aprons are heavy as they are made of lead, so the physician may not tolerate wearing one for long procedures. Lightweight alloy alternatives are a necessity as an increased number of physicians and technicians are required to wear aprons for longer time periods during more varied examinations. Non- lead protective aprons made of environment friendly, nontoxic, composite materials have been developed. Nonlead aprons consist of composite materials, mainly tungsten, bismuth, antimony and tin. They are 20% lighter than lead aprons.

Lead equivalence is measured by comparing the protection provided by pure lead sheet against that provided by the protective apron. Zero lead aprons refer to lead free apron.

Pregnant Radiation Worker

The NCRP (National Council on Radiological Protection and measurements) recommends that the dose to the fetus in pregnant radiation worker should not exceed 0.5 mSv per month. The ICRP recommends that the total dose to the abdomen of the mother should not exceed 2 mSv during entire pregnancy.

Ten-day rule: All females of reproductive age who need an X-ray examination should get it done within first 10 days of menstrual cycle to avoid irradiation of possible conception.

Radiography of area remote from fetus can be done safely at any time during pregnancy also by using protective lead apron, covering the fetus.

CHAPTER 39

Picture Archiving and Communication System

Picture archiving and communication system (PACS) stores and transmits images electronically over the internet or local area network (LAN) and viewed using suitable computer consoles and devices. The images can be accessed either within the hospital premises or at remote locations outside the hospital. PACS eliminates the need for maintaining hard copies of radiology films and reports by creating a filmless environment for easy and timely access to retrieve images and reports.

Radiology department has been a pioneer in developing PACS to its current high standards. In early 1980's the concept of using electronic storage and transmission of radiology images and reports was introduced. Due to prohibitive costs and technology issues PACS could not find many takers to start with. As the core technology of PACS rapidly progressed due to advances in technology, the capabilities of PACS improved potentially. For instance, the hard disk storage options improved, more images can be stored, retrieved and transmitted faster.

Presently PACS worldwide has become an indispensable workflow system in modern hospitals. Ideally CAT6 networking cables should be installed to maintain adequate transfer of data and images. Some hospitals continue to use outdated CAT5 networking cables; in such instances the PACS data transmission is slow. In addition to the networking cables appropriate routers, switches and firewalls are equally important for a secure and efficient network.

PICTURE ARCHIVING AND COMMUNICATION SYSTEM

The images of X-ray and fluoroscopy, diagnostic ultrasound, CT scan, MRI, mammography, PET scan and SPECT require:
- Secured network for transmission of patient information, preferably broadband internet.
- Workstations that have compatible hardware and software to retrieve the images and data for interpretation and reporting.
- Data storage archives on computer server to store images and reports.
- Server for backup copies at a remote location so that these images can be retrieved when the main PACS server is under maintenance care.

The PACS workflow system includes image acquisition; digital images are modified to PACS compatible images, data transfer to a central computer server, with appropriate data storage and archiving, remote access for viewing the images, providing support to clinicians. Some hospital might still use analogue radiographs that need to be scanned and converted into digital images for PACS. Its maintenance team should be readily available 24/7 to tackle software and hardware breakdown.

SOME TECHNICAL FEATURES OF PACS

- The hospital information system (HIS) server contains patient data and request for investigations (**Flowchart 1**), it is vendor specific (**Flowchart 2**), and should be compatible with PACS.

Section 2: Equipment, Physics and Procedures

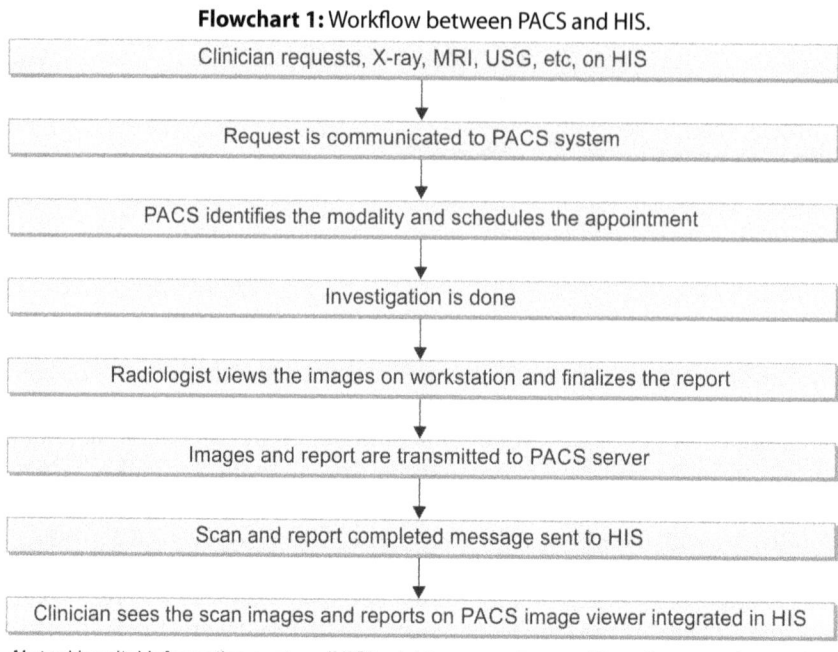

Flowchart 1: Workflow between PACS and HIS.

Note: Hospital information system (HIS) might use vendor specific software and operating system platform different from picture archiving and communication system (PACS)

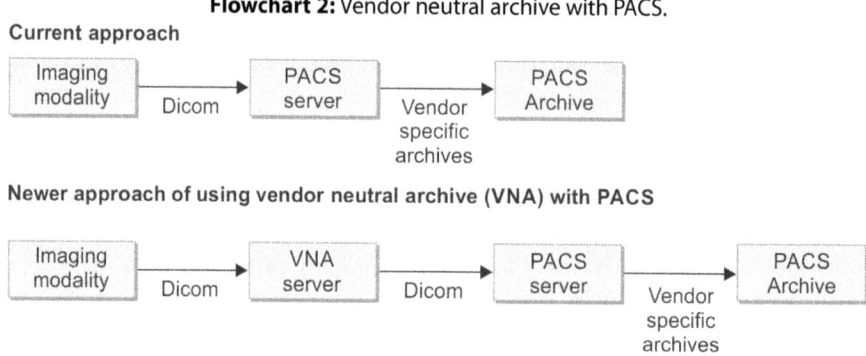

Flowchart 2: Vendor neutral archive with PACS.

- ❖ The Radiology Information System (RIS) contains the modality requested for **(Flowchart 3)**. This server is integrated with PACS.
- ❖ All the peripherals like external digital video decoders (DVD) writers, external universal serial bus (USB) ports, data backup and printing devices are integrated with PACS.
- ❖ Fine tuning of PACS with hospital digital imaging and communications in medicine (DICOM) is done for compressing images and reports, adjusting optimum speed of transmission, proxy IP (internet protocol) for networks, server functioning, remote data server for backups for image retrieval.
- ❖ PACS is a web-based system so it can be accessed wherever internet is available, it is hardware independent.
- ❖ Viewer can be installed on any operating systems like Linux, Mac or Windows for the radiologist to interpret them. PACS can support a wide range of mobile devices through

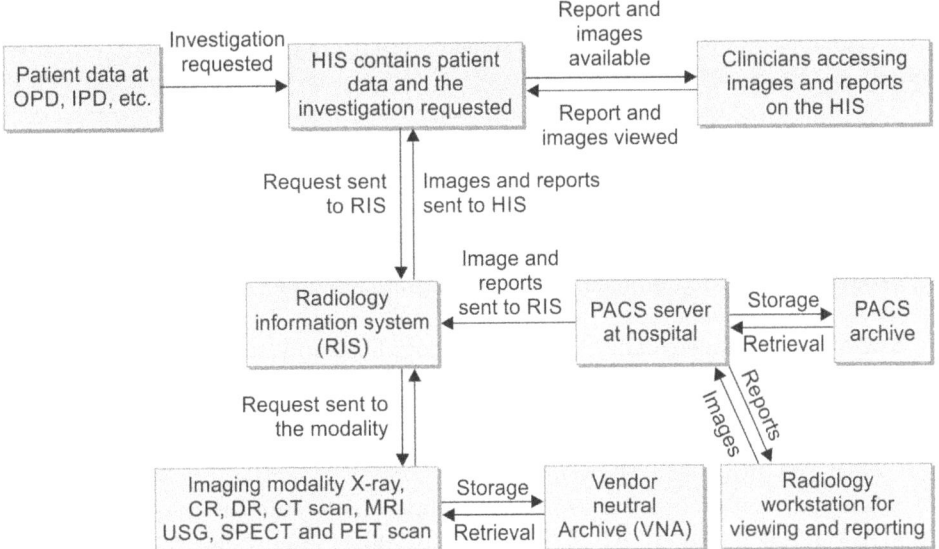

Flowchart 3: Radiology information system workflow.

Web Access to DICOM Objects (WADO) server. Mobile devices like iPhone, iPad, Android system-based phones and tablets are compatible with PACS.
* Voice recognition system is integrated in PACS which eliminates the manual transmission of reports with improve efficiency.
* The reporting formats and templates according to the HIS are uploaded on PACS. Digital signatures are available for reporting purposes. After a report has been saved and finalized the reporting software locks the report and no changes can be made. The report is then available for the clinicians.
* HL7 translator software integrates several PACS and radiology information systems. It is an interface ware that converts several formats from various sources to a standard format to view images and reports. It is more useful in Teleradiology to ensure compatibility between various PACS systems and helps to avoid errors. HL7 translator can improve the efficiency and serve as productivity enhancing tool.

Vendor Neutral Archive

PACS stores images in a vendor specific format of compression and storage, this can be a minor problem when the hospital decides to upgrade or switch to a newer PACS system. Vendor neutral archive (VNA) is a neutral format for storing the images directly from the imaging modality into the hospital computer server. Images are then transmitted from the VNA to PACS system. In this way, images can be stored in the hospital database and viewed/retrieved when necessary **(Flowchart 2)**.

Advantages of PACS

* Fast and easy access to images and reports in the hospital which improves patient care. Radiology images can be transmitted from peripheral clinics to hospitals for reporting the MRI, PET and CT scans due to lack of availability of radiologist at the clinic.

- No accumulation of paper reports and image films, PACS can store them electronically, saves time and space. This can prove cost-effective in the long-term planning.
- Images can be sent for second opinion/consultation using internet within the country and abroad.
- PACS can be connected to teleradiology software, radiologists can access the hospital PACS using their personal computers, iPads and mobile phones.

Drawbacks of PACS

- PACS is an expensive investment initially but the costs can be recovered over a 5-year-period.
- Important to train doctors, technicians, receptionists, other hospital staff to use PACS effectively.
- PACS eliminates the need for hard copy of radiology films and reports, the result is a filmless radiology department, this might take some time for the department to get used to this situation.
- Data might get lost due to some software or hardware problem. Storage of data at some remote location is very essential to retrieve the data.
- PACS has many different features and configurations to suit the unique needs of each hospital. Vendors try and promote their PACS products to hospitals. Some extra features quoted the vendors might not be required by the hospital. Ideally trial version of PACS should be installed for atleast a month in radiology department before any major decision is taken to purchase it.
- Radiology data images and reports might consume significant bandwidth of existing local area network (LAN) or internet traffic within the hospital. The PACS system selected should not overburden the existing networks in the hospital.
- Dedicated maintenance is needed to keep PACS operational. It involves addressing and overcoming issues related to widely varied networks, creating secure virtual private network tunnel, configuring multiple firewalls on network and testing digital imaging and communications in medicine (DICOM) transfers.

Training of Hospital Staff

On-site PACS training for hospital staff is essential to improve productivity and efficiency of PACS. Hospital staff should be given hands on training to make them comfortable using PACS systems. PACS can adapt to the unique requirements of different radiology departments. Ideally after the complete installation of PACS, the radiology department staff should be confident to compress images data and reports, transfer data efficiently so that productivity of PACS starts from the first day of installation. PACS vendors can also provide web-based updates and meetings to address issues regarding the usage of PACS similar to distance learning modules; interactive web sessions with periodic reviews are helpful.

Troubleshooting, Maintenance and Warranty Issues

Periodic troubleshooting, updating the software, installing new peripherals, server upgrades, retrieving lost files and regular maintenance checks ensure PACS functioning smoothly. Some examples include defragmentation of workstation memory, clearing the cache on workstations, updating antivirus software, clearing the computer registry. A dedicated and qualified PACS administrator with IT support team should be readily available at a short notice to resolve any glitches. The vendor should ideally provide warranty for the initial three years after installation of PACS. Annual renewal should be available at lower cost from fourth year onwards after installation. Any additional hardware upgrades or replacements for PACS server needs to be considered should also be taken into consideration as some radiology equipment might not be covered in warranty.

Changing or Switching to New PACS Vendor

The hospital might want to change to a new PACS vendor due to various reasons like obsolete software and hardware, requirement of the radiology department have changed, maintenance problems, etc. The transition to install a new PACS must be smooth and effective, also it is essential to training the staff all over again. There must be some specific features or functions in the new PACS which the existing PACS in the hospital cannot offer. It might be beneficial to discuss the problems faced in the new PACS with their existing customer base.

Quality Assurance in PACS

It is an essential aspect of PACS, from a clinical perspective. Image quality is important for any hospital using PACS. Basic system design and PACS training for staff can help to improve image quality. The quality of images viewed on PACS should be the same on different consoles used in hospital. The PACS images should in no way be inferior to hard copies of radiology images. PACS system has features to adjust the images for better viewing like contrast, brightness, flipping the image, zooming the image, add annotations and remarks to the images. Default settings can be applied to images so that each incoming images in PACS system are automatically optimized for viewing purposes. All PACS display devices such as computer consoles should undergo periodic quality assurance tests for monitoring PACS performance. If for some reason a PACS workstation does not meet all the requirements of the PACS, that machine should be labeled as non-suitable for PACS and explanation submitted to the hospital. PACS images that are not adequate for viewing should be kept in a separate folder in PACS so that they can be evaluated later by PACS maintenance team.

Computer Console Specifications

The LCD of computer console should operate at optimal resolution, this is to ensure that the ratio between screen pixels and screen resolution is 1:1 at all times.

Images where the image resolution is more than three megapixels are helpful in image interpretation.

PACS **(Fig. 1)** is a combination of hardware and software dedicated to short- and long-term storage, retrieval, management, distribution and presentation of images. The purpose of PACS is to improve efficiency by creating a filmless environment while maintaining or improving diagnostic ability of radiology department. PACS acts like an electronic gateway system using a dedicated PACS computer server. PACS uses both local area network (LAN) and internet, data management system that controls the workflow on a network and storage devices for image archives. The input of PACS can be from digital or analog sources, the input from analog sources are first converted into digital format before they can be sent to PACS system. Display devices for PACS-like computer consoles, voice dictation devices, keyboard and mouse are needed to view the images and data. The cost effectiveness of PACS must be proven before installing it in hospitals, initial setup is usually expensive. Training of radiology staff is important to effectively utilize PACS. Maintenance is done by a dedicated team of IT professionals. Switching or upgrading to a new vendor must be carefully done after weighting the pros and cons. VNA

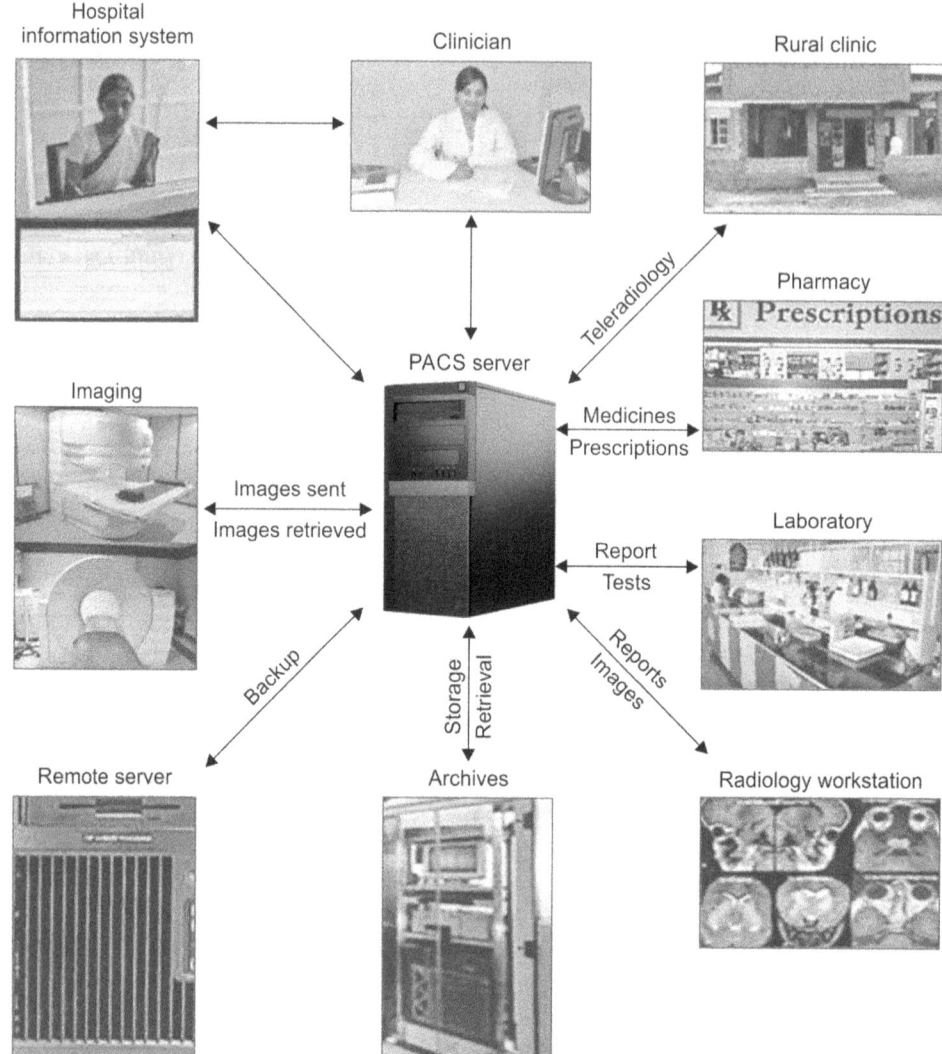

Fig. 1: PACS workflow.

can store images directly from the imaging modality and transmit the images to the PACS system. Quality assurance testing and monitoring is important to maintain image resolution for interpreting radiology images.

CHAPTER 40

Cloud Computing

The National Institute of Standards and Technology (NIST) has presented the clearest and most comprehensive definition of cloud computing. Cloud computing is a model for enabling convenient, on-demand network access to a shared pool of configurable computing resources which includes networks, servers, storage, applications and services, that can be rapidly provisioned and released with minimal management effort or service provider interaction. This cloud model promotes availability and is composed of essential characteristics, deployment models, and various service models. The institute categorizes cloud computing into 5 key categories—on-demand self-service, ubiquitous network access, location-independent resource pooling, rapid elasticity, and measured service. Cloud technologies can also be deployed as private, community, public, or hybrid clouds. Private clouds are operated for a specific organization, and are more popular in healthcare, whereas community clouds are shared by a number of organizations.

Cloud computing promotes the concept of "round-the-clock" radiology services, bedside radiology, point-of-care radiology, and instant radiology. It gives the technician, radiologists, physicians, and even patients the ability to review images on any display device with an internet connection. Cloud computing inserts flexibility which is necessary in a highly competitive and costly radiology practice. Cloud computing has the potential to transform a digital imaging practice and can further revolutionize the way we store, access, and process radiology data.

Radiology is increasingly dealing with large imaging data sets, complex algorithms, pre- and postprocessing requirements and an increasingly distributed environment. Distributed data grids perform much more efficiently compared to hard drives, primarily because memory is shared between data centers. Hence, performance is better. Deployments can also be more effectively and consistently managed across the healthcare enterprise, freeing users from the finer details of IT system configuration and maintenance, allowing them to focus instead on care delivery.

In this era of distributed digital imaging, there are specific needs for radiologists to have the ability not just to access images at the point of care, but also to be able to work efficiently and effectively from multiple locations, with full access to the complete imaging data sets, relevant priors, relevant clinical information, as well as to the right set of diagnostic tools from any location. Cloud-based deployments provide a more robust and sophisticated security strategy.

With digital revolution in radiology, it is resulting in more CDs and DVDs of patient studies than ever before. The future imaging department will have to deal a lot more intelligently with data and information explosion. With increase in the digital-imaging in healthcare, the data is growing from terabytes to petabytes in binary standard measurement (1 petabyte = 1000 terabytes; 1 terabyte = 1024 gigabytes; 1 gigabyte = 1024 megabytes, 1 megabyte = 1024 bytes). Cloud computing offers ways for these challenges, and knowledge of information systems, across healthcare enterprise.

CHAPTER 41

Photon-Counting Detector CT

Photon-counting CT or photon-counting detector CT (PCD-CT) is an emerging technology with the potential to dramatically change clinical CT. Photon-counting CT uses new energy-resolving X-ray detectors, with mechanisms that differ from conventional energy-integrating detectors. Photon-counting CT detectors count the number of incoming photons and measure photon energy. This technique results in higher contrast-to-noise ratio, improved spatial resolution and optimized spectral imaging.

Photon-counting CT reduces radiation exposure, increased spatial resolution, correction of beam-hardening artifacts, reconstruct images at a higher resolution and optimize the use of contrast agents, and create opportunities for quantitative imaging relative to current CT technology.

A photon counting detector is made from a semiconducting material that allows for the direct conversion of the X-ray photon to an electrical signal. In this case, the many photons hitting the detector can be counted individually, enabling a more accurate signal to generate images.

Photon counting is a technique in which individual photons are counted using a single-photon detector (SPD). A single-photon detector emits a pulse of signal for each detected photon.

Photon-counting CT improves on conventional CT because the X-ray photon is converted directly to electrons. Photon-counting CT is very fast, a single pulse takes just about 10 nanoseconds and with fast electronics, each X-ray is measured providing superior resolution.

Photon-counting CT angiogram allows for significant reduction of contrast medium and radiation dose while maintaining good to excellent image quality.

Photon-counting CT with improved spatial resolution and spectral reconstructions, yielding advantages for cardiac, vascular, thoracic and musculoskeletal CT imaging.

CHAPTER 42

CT Technologist Questions/Answers

Common CT technologist questions with answers for better understanding of the subject, as well as for practical examination and placement interviews.

Q.1. What is the importance of patient positioning in CT scans?

Ans. Patient positioning is of utmost importance in CT scans as accurate positioning ensures that the area of interest is properly captured within the scan field, providing the radiologist with clear and precise images for diagnosis. Misaligned positioning can lead to suboptimal image quality or even missed pathology, which may require additional imaging or result in incorrect diagnoses.

Proper patient positioning helps minimize radiation exposure by ensuring that only the targeted area is exposed to the X-ray beam. This is particularly important when scanning sensitive areas such as the head or chest, where minimizing radiation dose is critical.

Q.2. What is the difference between axial and helical scanning?

Ans. In axial scanning, the CT scanner acquires images slice while the patient table moves incrementally between each rotation of the X-ray tube and detectors. After each complete rotation, the table stops momentarily to acquire an image before moving on to the next position. This process is time-consuming and may result in gaps or overlaps between slices.

Whereas helical scanning or spiral or volumetric scanning, involves continuous rotation of the X-ray tube and detectors around the patient while the table moves smoothly through the gantry. This allows for faster acquisition of data and generates a more seamless set of images without any gaps or overlaps. Helical scanning has become the preferred method in modern CT scanners due to its efficiency, improved image quality, and ability to reconstruct images in multiple planes using post-processing techniques.

Q.3. How to ensure that radiation exposure to patients is minimized during a CT scan?

Ans. To minimize radiation exposure during a CT scan, one must adhere to the ALARA (As Low As Reasonably Achievable) principle.

Before performing a scan, review the patient's medical history to determine the appropriate examination parameters, tube current, voltage, and slice thickness based on the patient's size and the specific diagnostic requirements.

Application of dose reduction technique, i.e., automatic exposure control (AEC) to adjust radiation output in real-time according to the patient's anatomy.

Ensure proper patient positioning and use of shielding devices to protect sensitive areas from unnecessary radiation exposure. Also maintain communication with patients throughout the process, providing reassurance to help them remain still, which can reduce the need for repeat scans due to motion artifacts. These practices collectively contribute to minimizing radiation exposure while.

Q.4. What are some common artifacts seen on CT images and how can they be reduced or eliminated?

Ans. Common artifacts seen in CT images are beam hardening, motion artifacts, and metal artifacts. Beam hardening occurs when lower-energy X-rays are absorbed by the patient's body, causing a streaking effect on the image. This artifact can be reduced by software-based correction algorithms or increase the tube voltage to produce higher-energy X-rays.

Motion artifacts result from patient movement during scanning, which can cause blurring effects on the image. To minimize these artifacts, patient is instructed to remain still, use immobilization devices if require and employ faster scan times to reduce the chance of movement during the acquisition process.

Metal artifacts occur due to the presence of metallic objects within the patient's body, such as dental fillings or implants, which create streaks and dark bands on the image. To address this issue, we can utilize metal artifact reduction (MAR) algorithms available in modern CT scanners or adjust the scanning parameters, such as increasing the kVp or using iterative reconstruction techniques.

Above strategies help improve image quality.

Q.5. Explain the process of image reconstruction in CT imaging.

Ans. This question seeks to assess your understanding of the technical aspects of your role as a CT technologist. Image reconstruction is a vital component of CT technology, as it involves converting raw data from the CT scan into a format that can be visualized and interpreted by medical professionals. Demonstrating your knowledge of this process shows that you are well-versed in the underlying principles of CT imaging and can effectively operate the equipment to provide accurate diagnostic information.

Image reconstruction transforms raw data collected during scanning into interpretable images. The process begins with the acquisition of data, where X-ray beams pass through the patient's body and are detected by an array of detectors on the opposite side. This generates attenuation profiles for each slice at various angles as the gantry rotates around the patient.

The next step involves using mathematical algorithms to reconstruct these attenuation profiles into cross-sectional images. One common method is filtered back-projection (FBP), which essentially reverses the path of the X-rays and compiles the projections onto a grid representing the image plane. Another approach is iterative reconstruction, which uses optimization techniques to minimize discrepancies between measured and calculated projections iteratively.

These reconstructed images can then be further processed and analyzed to diagnose medical conditions. As a CT technologist, understanding this process helps to optimize scan parameters and ensure high-quality images.

Q.6. What safety measures are required while injecting intravenous contrast?

Ans. Administering intravenous contrast can result in risks like allergic reactions or kidney damage, so it is essential to understand the proper protocols and procedures to minimize these risks and effectively respond to any adverse reactions that may occur.

Review the patient's medical history and inquire about any allergies or previous reactions to contrast agents. This helps me identify potential risks and determine if premedication is necessary.

Ensure proper IV placement and use the appropriate injection rate based on the patient's condition and the specific contrast agent being used.

Monitor the patient throughout the procedure for any signs of adverse reactions, such as difficulty breathing, swelling, or hives.

Q.7. How to handle patients who may have claustrophobia or anxiety for undergoing a CT scan?

Ans. Handling patients with claustrophobia or anxiety is an inevitable part of the job. Interviewers want to know how well you can manage such situations, ease the patient's concerns, and provide a comfortable environment for them during the CT scan. Your ability to handle patients with special needs reflects your level of professionalism and your dedication to quality patient care.

When dealing with claustrophobia or anxiety focus should be to create a comfortable and reassuring environment by explaining the procedure and answering their questions patiently to build trust and lessen their fears.

In severe cases, mild sedation is given to ensure patient's well-being during the procedure.

Q.8. What steps are followed for proper infection control in CT suite?

Ans. For infection control in the CT suite, technician to ensure patient safety and prevent cross-contamination.

He should make sure that the equipment is cleaned and disinfected according to manufacturer guidelines and institutional policies. This involves wiping down surfaces with appropriate disinfectant solutions between patients and performing more thorough cleaning at regular intervals.

He should follow hand hygiene protocols by washing hands thoroughly before and after each patient interaction, as well as using gloves when necessary.

Contaminated materials, such as used gloves and other disposable items in designated biohazard containers. He should stay updated on any changes in infection control guidelines and participate in ongoing training to ensure best practices are consistently followed within the CT suite.

Q.9. What are the differences between single-slice and multi-slice CT scanners?

Ans. Single-slice CT scanners are with single-detector row, it acquires one image slice per rotation. Single-slice CT scanning process is slow and cost of equipment is comparatively less.

Multi-slice CT scanners has multiple rows of detectors that allow to capture multiple slices simultaneously during each rotation. This results in faster scan, better image resolution. They are essential for perfusion and angiographic studies.

Through the process of scanning, technician should maintain communication with the radiologist to ensure that the selected parameters align with their diagnostic needs. He should adhere to established guidelines and protocols. This will ensures high-quality images that facilitate accurate diagnoses while prioritizing patient safety and comfort.

Q.10. Any serious emergency encountered during a CT scan.

Ans. Allergic reaction to the contrast agent is a serious emergency encountered during a CT scan on patient showing any sign of distress and difficulty breathing, the injection of contrast or the scan is immediately stopped and follow the institutional emergency protocol. In most institutions Code Blue is alerted.

Even before code blue comes into action, oxygen is administered and vital signs are monitored.

Q.11. How to manage trauma or critical care patients for CT scan?

Ans. To manage trauma or critical care patients time factor is important, they require immediate imaging, prioritization, teamwork and effective communication.

During the scanning process, technician works in close association with the radiologists and healthcare professionals to provide accurate and timely results.

Q.12. How to minimize motion artifacts in CT images?

Ans. Minimizing motion artifacts is essential for obtaining high-quality CT images and accurate diagnosis by use is effective patient communication, which involves explaining the importance of remaining still during the scan and providing clear instructions on breathing techniques. It also involves proper patient positioning and immobilization using available devices like straps or cushions when needed.

Q.13. How to ensure patient privacy and confidentiality?

Ans. Patient privacy and confidentiality is maintained by discussing patient information in areas where conversations cannot be overheard by unauthorized individuals.

Medical records and images are kept secure and ensure that digital files are password-protected and accessible only to authorized personnel.

Q.14. What is difference between HRCT and routine CT scan?

Ans. High-resolution computed tomography (HRCT) is done to enhance image resolution. It is used in the diagnosis, most commonly for lung disease, assessing the lung parenchyma.

In routine CT scans of lungs, 3 to 5 millimeter slices are done for evaluation. These slices are good for nodules or masses but for appreciating the fine details HRCT scans with one millimeter thickness slices are taken. The thinner slices allow for a much more detailed analysis of lung parenchyma.

HRCT is also done for temporal bone. HRCT of the temporal bone is used to diagnose various middle ear diseases such as otitis media and cholesteatoma.

Index

Page numbers followed by *f* refer to figure, *fc* refer to flowchart, and *t* refer to table.

A

Abdomen 50, 107
 axial CT section of 51*f*-58*f*
 CT of 51*f*
 plain X-ray of 129*f*
Abdominal angiography, CT of 121*f*
Absorbed dose 140
 quantity of 140
Acetabular notch, level of 78*f*
Acetabulum 76
Adrenal glands 60
Advanced slip ring technology 96
Adverse reactions, treatment of 117
Agger nasi 23
Air 115
Airway 111
 edema 118
Albuterol 118
Aluminium 99
Anal canal 55, 60*f*
Analog-to-digital conversion of signal 97
Anaphylactic reactions, treatment of 117
Anatomical planes 3
Anesthesia, under local 132
Aneurysm, suspicion of 130*f*
Angiographic catheters 132*f*
Angiography, CT of 121
Angulation artifact 123, 123*f*
Ankle joint 76
Annular pancreas 53
Antimony 145
Aorta, descending 130*f*
Aortic reconstruction 130*f*
Appendix, axial CT section of 61*f*
Arachnoiditis 120
Arch of aorta, level of 44*f*
 branches of 43*f*
Artery, left anterior descending 46
Arthrography 115
Artifact 123
 partial volume 124, 125*f*
Artificial intelligence 89
Arytenoid cartilage, level of 27*f*
Asthma 121
Atomic energy regulatory board 90, 143

Auditory canal, external 17
Auditory ossicles 17
Automatic exposure control 155
AV node 46*f*
Axial scanning 155
Axial typical vertebra (C3-C7) volume 33*f*
Azygos vein 45*f*

B

Barium sulfate formulations, hypersensitivity to 116
Basal ganglia 6
 level of 9*f*
Basilar artery 12
Biconvex extradural hematoma 130
 right 130*f*
Bilateral maxillary hemosinus 109*f*
Biliary duct stones, percutaneous removal of 135
Binary standard measurement 153
Biopsy 134*f*
Biopsy
 CT guided 113
 precision 134
 posterior approach 135*f*
Bismuth 145
Blood vessels, abnormal 133
Body of mandible and frontal bone, fracture of 109*f*
Bone 111
 frontal 109
 high frontal 11*f*
 partial volume of 125*f*
Bony labyrinth, wall of 17
Bradycardia 116
Brain 5, 6
 anatomically 5
 axial CT section of 7*f*-10*f*
 CT scan of 4*f*
 embryologically 5
 plain CT of 130*f*
Breast 142
Bronchi, level of 39*f*
Bronchial circulation 37
Bronchial tree 110
Bronchospasm 118
 mild 118
Buccal mucosa 24

C

C1 vertebra 30f
C1-C2 coronal reconstruction 31f
C2 vertebra 31f
Calcaneum
    bone 84f
    level of 83f
Calcium
    borate 126
    fluoride 126
    sulfate 126
Calculus, large 129
Calvarium 6
Carbon dioxide 115
Cardiac CT imaging 154
Cardiac disease 121
Cardiac masses 46
Cardinal ligament 63
Cardiovascular reactions 117
Carina, level of 39f
C-arm frame 94
Carotid artery, internal 12
Carpel bones
    level of distal row of 73f
    proximal row of 74f
Cartilages 76
Catheter 132, 133
    and sheaths 132f
Cathode 91
Cells, proliferation of 142
Centrum semiovale, level of 9f
Cerebellar artery
    anterior inferior 12
    superior 12
Cerebellum 6
    level of 7f
Cerebral artery
    anterior 12
    middle 12
    posterior 12
Cerebral hemisphere, level of entire 9f
Cerebrospinal fluid 6
Cervical vertebra 33
    (C3-C7), typical 32f
Chamberlain line 29
Chest 37, 107
    apices, axial CT section 38f
    axial CT section 39f, 40f, 41, 42f-45f
    in mediastinal window, axial CT section of 44f, 45f
    wall 42
    window settings for 38
Cholesteatoma 158
Circle of Willis 11, 12f
    arteries forming 11
Claustrophobia 157
Cloud computing 153
Cobra 132f
Code blue 136
Collateral ligaments 76
Collimation 99
Collimators 99
Colon 57f
    descending 55
    obstruction of 116
Common artifacts 156
Common interventional radiology procedures 132
Communicating artery
    anterior 12
    posterior 12
Communication
    maintain 155
    system 104, 147
Complex vascular structures, analysis of 110
Computed tomography 132
    contrast 114
    number scale 105
    room 145
    sixth generation 136
    technologist 88
    triple-phase 136
Computed tomography images
    artificial intelligence on 89
    diagnosis on 128
    principles of 156
    vascular 154
Computed tomography scan 103, 138, 138t, 155, 157
    hardware 100
    installation of 90
    pitch in 136
    technologist 88
    tidbits on 136
    unit 100f
Computed tomography scanner
    components of 100
    highest slice 136
    newest 137
    single-slice 157
Computed tomography system
    first generation 93, 94f
    generations of 93
    second generation 94f
    third generation 95f
Computer console specifications 151
Console 100, 103
Contiguous slices, series of 106
Continuous helical scan 96
Conventional protective aprons 145
Converts electronic energy 91
Copper, made of 99
Coronal plane 3
    posterior 122f
Coronal view (C2-C4 level) volume 34f

Coronary artery 46, 46f, 47f, 122f
   left 49
   main 46
   right 49
Cosmic radiation 141
Couinaud classification 50f
Cranial fossae
   anterior 5
   middle 5
   posterior 5
Craniovertebral junction 29
Cremasteric artery 60
Cricoid cartilage, level of 27f
Critical care patients 158
Cross-sectional high-resolution images 121
Crystal lattice structure act 126
Cuboid bone 84f
Curved plane reconstructions 111
Cystic duct, normal 53

D

Dark field computed tomography 136
Data acquisition system 97
Deep learning
   post-processing 89
   reconstruction 136
Delayed reactions 117
Detecting voxels 110
Detector-data ring mismatch 123
Deterministic effects 141
Diaphragm, level of 42f
Diatrizoate 114
Digital imaging and communications in medicine 148
   transfers 150
Digital signatures 149
Digital subtraction angiography, guidance of 132
Digital video decoders 148
Dilatations 111
Diminished organ function 141
Distal femur, level of 79f
Distal radioulnar joints 64
Dominant coronary artery 49
Dose
   limitation 143
   reduction technique, application of 155

E

Ear
   diseases, middle 158
   external 16
   inner 16, 18
   middle 16, 17
Elbow
   axial CT section of 68f-70f
   coronal CT recon of 71f
   sagittal CT recon of 71f, 72f

Elbow joint 64
   coronal CT recon of 70f
   CT of 68
Electron 91
   deceleration of 91
   orbital shells 141
Electronic medical record 139
   usage of 139
Endodermal diverticulum, second 53
Epidural space 6
Epiglottis, level of 25f
Epinephrine 118
Ethmoid bulla 23
Ethmoid sinuses
   anterior 19
   posterior 19
Ethmoidal air cells 23
Extradural space 6
Extravasation 117
   injuries 119
Eyeball 12

F

Face 24
Feldspar 126
Female pelvis, axial CT section of 59f-61f
Femoral condyles, level of 79f
Femoral head 76
Femur
   head of 77f
   level of proximal shaft of 77f
Fibula 81f
   level of
      intercondylar eminence of 81f
      proximal part of 80f
Filament cathode 91
Filtered back-projection method 98
Filtration 99
Fissure 50
Floor of mouth 24
Fluid drainages 113
Flu-like symptoms, development of 117
Fluoroscopic computed tomography 113
Fluoroscopy, CT of 113
Focus film distance 92
Foot
   and ankle joint 76
      CT sections of 82
   axial CT section of 82f, 83f
   sagittal CT recon of 84f
Foramen
   lacerum 5
   magnum 5
   of Winslow 58
   ovale 5
   rotundum 5
   spinosum 5

Forearm 64
Forebrain 5
Fourth generation system 95, 96f
Fourth ventricle, level of 7f
Fovea, level of 77f
Fracture 109

G

Gallbladder 52
   and pancreas, level of middle of 55f
   normal 52
Gantry tilt 136
Gastrografin 115
Gastrointestinal system 54
Gastrointestinal tract 115
   perforation 116
Gastropancreatic ligament 58
Gastrophrenic ligament 57, 58
General radiation protection 99
Gerota fascia 128f
Gingiva 24
Glenohumeral joint 66f
Glottis 25
Gonadal artery 61
Gonadal veins 61
Good anatomical knowledge 88
Great toe 76

H

H_1 antihistamines 118
Hair loss 141
Haller cell 23
Hand 64
   3D recon of 75f
Hard palate 24
Head
   and neck 107
   in bone window, axial CT section of 10f, 11f
   of humerus, level middle part of 65f
Headhunter 132f
Health effects 141
Healthcare
   centers, manages 139
   skills 88
Heart 46, 47f
   chambers of 45f
   imaging methods 46
   in coronal plane 47f
Helical scanning 155
Hemiazygos vein 45f
Hepatic vein
   branches 135
   left 50
Hepatoduodenal ligament 57
Higher density enables 110
High-quality images 157

Hilum, level of 40f
Hindbrain 5
Hip
   axial CT section of 77f
   coronal CT reconstruction of 78f
Hip joint 76
   CT sections of 77
   level of 77f
   superior part of 78f
HL7 translator 149
Hospital information system 147
   workflow 148fc
Hospital staff, training of 150
Hounsfield scale 104
Hounsfield units 38, 104
Hounsfield value 38
Human body, organs of 87
Humeroradial articulation 71f, 71f
Humeroulnar joint 71f
Humerus
   head of 66f
   level distal shaft of 68f
   level epicondyles of 69f
   part of shaft of 66f
   superior part of head of 65f
   supracondylar ridge of 68f
Hypopharynx 25
   level of 26f
Hypotension 116
Hysterosalpingography 115

I

Idiosyncratic reactions 116
Iliac arteries, aortic bifurcation into 58f
Image processor 103
Image reconstruction 88, 106
Infection control 157
Inflammation 116
Infraspinatus 64
Intensity projection, minimum 110
Interalveolar septum 37
Interlobular septa 37
Internal circuits 101
Interventional radiology 132
   principle of 132
Intestine, large 55
Intrathecal administration 114
Intravascular iodinated agent arterial opacification 115
Intravenous contrast, injecting 156
Intravenous insertion 88
Iodinated contrast media, adverse reactions to 115
Iodinated intravascular agents 114
Iodine 114
Iodixanol 114
Iohexol 114
Iomeron 114

Ionic dimer 114
Ionic monomers 114
Ionizing radiation 138
Iopamidol 114
Iothalamate 114
Iotrolan 114
Ioxaglate 114

J

Jaundice 134
Jugular foramen 5
Jugular vein, level of internal 43*f*

K

Kidneys 56*f*, 59
  level of
    middle of both 55*f*
    upper pole of both 54*f*
Knee
  axial CT section of 79*f*, 80*f*
  coronal CT recon of 80*f*, 81*f*
  volume rendered 3D CT recon of 82*f*
Knee joint 76, 81*f*
  CT section of 79

L

Laryngeal edema 118
  mild-to-moderate 118
Laryngospasm 118
Larynx 25
Lateral ventricles, level of 8*f*
Lead equivalence 145
Lead free aprons 145
Left temporal bone, axial CT section of 16*f*-18*f*
Lens 12
Leukemias 142
Ligament
  broad 59*f*, 62, 63
  uterosacral 63
Lingual lobe 41*f*
Lingular segments, level of 40*f*
Linux 148
Lip 24
Lithium
  borate 126
  fluoride 126
Liver 50
  anatomy of 50
    classification of 50
  inferior portion of 50
  level of 45*f*, 53*f*
  normal 52
  segments 50*f*-52*f*
Lobe
  high frontal 10*f*
  lower 41*f*, 42*f*
  middle 40*f*, 41*f*
Local area network 151
Lower extremity 76
  joints of 76
Lower lobe, level of apical segments of 41*f*
Lumbar vertebra 33
  typical 36*f*
Lumbosacral region 33
Lung
  apex 43*f*
  carcinoma of 142
  interstitium of 37
  right 37, 134*f*
  segmental division of 37
  window 38, 38*f*-42*f*
Lymph nodes, enlarged 42

M

Mac 148
MaCkenrodt ligament 63
Magnetic resonance imaging scan 138, 138*t*
Maintenance and warranty issues 150
Male pelvis, axial CT section of 62*f*
Mammography 91
Materials exhibiting thermoluminescence 126
Maxillary sinuses 19
  level of 24*f*
  level superior part of 24*f*
Maximum intensity projection 110
  displays 110
Mediastinal structures 42
Mediastinal window 42-44*f*
Mediastinum 37
  CT of 43
  window settings for 38
Medical records 139, 158
  hard copy of 139
  keeping 139
Meninges 6
Meningiomas 142
Mesencephalon 5
Mesenchymal cells 53
Mesenteric artery, superior 54
Metacarpal, level of bases of 73*f*
Metal artifacts 156
Metallic clips 123
Metallic implant 123
Metallic stents, self-expanding 133
Metallic Thomas splint 124*f*
Metaproterenol inhaler 118
Metrizoate 114
Midbrain 5
Modern computed tomography systems 101
Molybdenum 91
Motion artifact 123, 124*f*, 156
  minimize 158

Multiplanar reconstructions 111
Multiplanar reformatting 106
Multiply radiation absorbed dose 140
Multislice CT scanners 157
Multislice spiral CT 97
Muscles 76
Musculoskeletal computed tomography imaging 154
Myelography
   advantages of 120
   CT of 120
Myocardium 46

N

Nasal cavity 19
National Institute of Standards and Technology 153
Nausea 141
Neck 24
   axial CT section of 24*f*-28*f*
Needle 132
   biopsy 133
Nephropathy 116
Nephrostomy placement 133
Newer picture archiving and communications systems 149
   vendor 151
Nonidiosyncratic reactions 116
Nonionic dimer 114
Nonionic monomers 114
Non-linear course 110
Normal coronary angiography, CT of 46

O

Oblique coronal plane 48*f*
Occipital artery 5
Occipital condyle 30*f*
Onodi cells 23
Ophthalmic veins 15
Optic nerve 15
Optimized protection 143
Oral contrast 115
Orbit 5, 12
Orbital fissure, inferior 15
Organic iodine compounds 114
Osmolar contrast media, high 115
Osteosarcomas 142
Ostiomeatal unit 19
Otitis media 158

P

Pancreas 53, 128*f*
   body of 55*f*
   head of 56*f*
   uncinate process of 56*f*
Pancreatic duct 53
Pancreatitis 128

Para-aortic lymph node, left 135*f*
Paranasal sinuses 19
   axial CT section of 19*f*-21*f*
   coronal CT recon of 22*f*
   sagittal CT
      recon of 22*f*
      reconstruction of 23*f*
Parathyroid glands 28
Paraxial planes 106
Parenchyma 111
Parenchymal interstitial
   edema 128*f*
   interstitium 37
Parenchymal necrosis 128*f*
Parotid gland 28
Patella 80*f*
   level of 79*f*
Pathologic spine conditions 120
Patient care 88
Patient table 100, 102
Patient waiting area 145
Pelvic ligaments 63
Pelvic muscles 60*f*
Pelvis 50, 76
   axial CT section of 58*f*, 59*f*
Pencil beam scan 94*f*
Penile anatomy 62*f*
Percutaneous biliary duct drainage 134
Pericardium 46
Perirenal fat 128*f*
Peritoneum, layers of 58
Personnel shielding 145
Pharyngeal artery 5
Phosphor crystal 126
Photon
   detectors 102
   number of 126
Photon-counting
   CT 154
      angiogram 154
   detector CT 154
Phrenicocolic ligament 58
Picture archiving and communication system 148*fc*
   advantages of 149
   drawbacks of 150
   quality assurance in 151
   technical features of 147
   workflow 148*fc*, 152*f*
Picture archiving system 147
Pituitary gland 6
   level of 7*f*
Portal vein
   branches 135
   left 50
   level of 54*f*
   right 50, 52
Posterior oblique coronal plane 47*f*, 122*f*
Post-patient collimators 99

Potassium bromide 126
Pouch of Douglas, rectouterine 62
Pregnant radiation worker 146
Prosencephalon 5
Prostate 61, 62f
Protective lead apron 146
Proximal metacarpal, level of 72f
Pulmonary artery 37
  level of main 44f
Pulmonary circulation 37
  primary 37
Pulmonary veins 46
Pyloric stenosis 116

R

Radiation
  absorbed dose 140
  effects 141
    classification of 141
  environment 145
  exposure 126, 142, 155
  hazards 141
  high levels of 141
  poisoning 141
  safety 88
  sickness 141
  type of 90, 140
  units 140
Radiation protection 143
  actions, triad of 144
  objective of 143
  principles of 143
Radio-capitellum joint 72f
Radiofrequency energy 138
Radiography 87
Radiology
  department 147
  images, transmission of 147
  information system 148
    workflow 149fc
  technologist 88
Radioulnar joint, proximal 70f
Radius 74f
  level head of 69f
  level proximal shaft of 70f
Ranitidine 118
Rectal biopsy, recent 116
Rectum 55
  neoplastic lesions of 116
Renal arteries 60
Renal condition 121
Renal cysts, bilateral 106f
Renal veins, level of 56f
Retroperitoneal fat necrosis 128f
Retroperitoneum 60
Retrosternal region 37
Rhombencephalon 5

Right hand, accidental motion of 123
Right orbit
  axial CT section of 12f, 13f
  coronal CT recon of 14f
  sagittal CT recon of 14f
Ring artifact 123f
Robotic assistance biopsy 134
Roentgen equivalent man 140
Room shielding 144
Round ligament 63
Round-the-clock radiology services, concept of 153

S

S1 coronal recon 36f
S1 vertebra 36f
Sacroiliac joints 36f
Sacroiliac region 33
Sagittal view (C2-C4 level) volume 34f
Salivary glands 28
  pairs of 28
Scalp 6
Scanning unit 100, 101
Scatter radiation artifact 94
Second generation system 94
Selective angiography, pigtail for 132f
Server contains patient data 147
Shaded surface display 111
Shielding 144
Shoulder
  axial CT section of 65f, 66f
  coronal recon of 66f
  CT of 65
  volume rendered 3D recon of 67f
Shoulder joint 64
  sagittal recon of 67f
Sickness, diagnosis of 87
Sidewinder 132f
Sievert 140
Sigmoid colon 55, 59f
Single breath hold 96
Single-photon detector 154
Sinus
  frontal 19
  walls of 109
Skills, mandatory 112
Skin 142
  burns 141
Skull
  base 5
  level of base of 10f
  table 6
Slice thickness 136
Slip-ring technology 97
Small bowel loops 58f
Small intestine 55
  obstructing lesions of 116

Soft palate 24
Soft tissue 76, 107
    contrast 121
Sphenoid
    sinus 19
    wing of 12
Spinal artery, anterior 12
Spinal cord, coverings of 29
Spinal fluid and seizure, leakage of 120
Spinal needle 120
Spine 108
Spleen 53
    level of 53*f*
Splenic flexure 55
Splenogonadal fusion 53
Splenorenal ligament 58
Staghorn calculi right kidney 129
Stenosis 111
Stochastic effects 141, 142
Stomach, level of 53*f*
Streak artifact 124*f*
Styloid processes, level of 74*f*
Subpleural connective tissue 37
Subscapularis 64
Suprahyoid portion, deep spaces of 26
Suprarenal glands 60
Supraspinatus 64
Surrounding tissue 110
Symmetric hyperdensities 124
Synovial joint, type of 76

T

T12-L1 coronal 35*f*
Talus, level of 83*f*
Tarsal bones 84*f*
    level of 82*f*
Temporal bone 16
Temporal lobes, level of 8*f*
Ten-day rule 146
Testicular artery 60
Thermoluminescent dosimeter 126, 126*f*, 127
    advantages of 127
Third generation system 95
Third ventricle, level of 8*f*
Thomas splint, right thigh in 124*f*
Thoracic aorta 37, 46, 130*f*
    aneurysm, large descending 131
    level of
        ascending 44*f*
        descending 44*f*
Thoracic CT imaging 154
Thoracic spine 33
Thoracic vertebra 35*f*
    typical 33, 34*f*, 35*f*
Thoracolumbar junction 33

Three-dimensional imaging 109
Thymic cyst, diagnosis of 134*f*
Thyroid 142
    cartilage, level of 26*f*
    conditions 121
    gland 28
Tibia 81
    and fibula, level of distal shaft of 82*f*
    intercondylar eminence of 80*f*
    level of proximal part of 80*f*
Tin 145
Tissue sample, biopsy of 132
Tongue, base of 24
Tonsillar region 24
Tortuous thoracic aorta 130
Tracheobronchial tree 37
Transjugular intrahepatic portosystemic stent 135
Transverse colon 55
    peritoneal spaces below 57
    with haustra 57*f*
Transverse plane 3
Trauma, manage 158
Trazograf 115
Trigeminal nerve, branches of 15
Troubleshooting 150
Tungsten 145
    anode 91

U

Ulna 74*f*
    level proximal shaft of 70*f*
Unilocular cystic lesion 133*f*
Unresponsive patient 118
Upper arm 64
Upper extremity, joints of 64
Urethra 60*f*
    male 61
Urinary bladder diverticulum 129
Urogenital system 59
Urticaria 118
Uterus 59*f*
Uvula, level of 25*f*

V

Vaginal introitus 61*f*
Vascular defects 111
Vasovagal reactions 116
Vault of skull, all bones of 11*f*
Vendor neutral archive 148*fc*, 149
Vertebral artery 12
Vertebral canal 29
Vertebral column 29
Vessels 111
Virtual endoscopy 111

Vocal cords 25
   level of true 27f
Volumetric data, acquisition of 106
Volumetric rendering techniques 110

W

Weakness 141
Window 137, 148
   level 38, 107
   narrow 107
   setting 107
   wide 107
   width 38, 107
Women radiation workers 145
Wrist 64
   axial CT section of 72f-74f
   CT of 72
   joint 64
   three D recon of 75f

X

X-ray
   absorption, element for 114
   equipment 141
   examination room 144
   generator 101
   production of 91, 91f
   room 145
   shielding elements 102
   tube 101
      inherent filtration of 99
      shielding 144
XY coordinate 110

Z

Zero lead aprons 145

EU GSPR Authorised Reprsentative
Logos Europe, 9 rue Nicolas Poussin
1700, La Rochelle, France
Phone: +33 (0) 6 67 93 73 78
E-mail: contact@logoseurope.eu

www.ingramcontent.com/pod-product-compliance
Ingram Content Group UK Ltd.
Pitfield, Milton Keynes, MK11 3LW, UK
UKHW050457150426
5217IPUK00025B/1720